Juicing:

The Ultimate Juicing & Smoothie Guide for Weight Loss, Vibrant Energy & Better Health Without Grueling Workouts

Copyright Notice

No part of this book may be reproduced or transmitted in any form whatsoever, electronic, or mechanical, including photocopying, recording, or by any information storage or retrieval system without expressed written, dated and signed permission from the author. All copyrights are reserved.

Disclaimer

Reasonable care has been taken to ensure that the information presented in this book is accurate. However, the reader should understand that the information provided does not constitute legal, medical or professional advice of any kind.

No Liability: this product is supplied "as is" and without warranties. All warranties, express or implied, are hereby disclaimed. Use of this product constitutes acceptance of the "No Liability" policy. If you do not agree with this policy, you are not permitted to use or distribute this product.

We shall not be liable for any losses or damages whatsoever (including, without limitation, consequential loss or damage) directly or indirectly arising from the use of this product.

Claim your FREE Audiobook Now

Autoimmune Healing Transform Your Health, Reduce Inflammation, Heal the Immune System and Start Living Healthy

Do you have an overall sense of not feeling your best, but it has been going on so long that it's actually normal to you?

If you answered yes to any of these question, you may have an autoimmune disease.

Autoimmune diseases are one of the ten leading causes of death for women in all age groups and they affect nearly 25 million Americans.

In fact millions of people worldwide suffer from autoimmunity whether they know it or not.

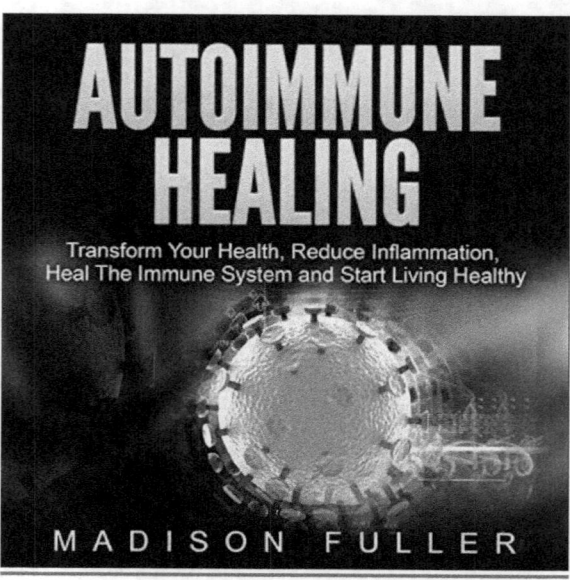

Free Newsletter

Health, longevity and lifestyle tips and advice

Sign up to get the exclusive Madison Fuller e-newsletter, sent out every week

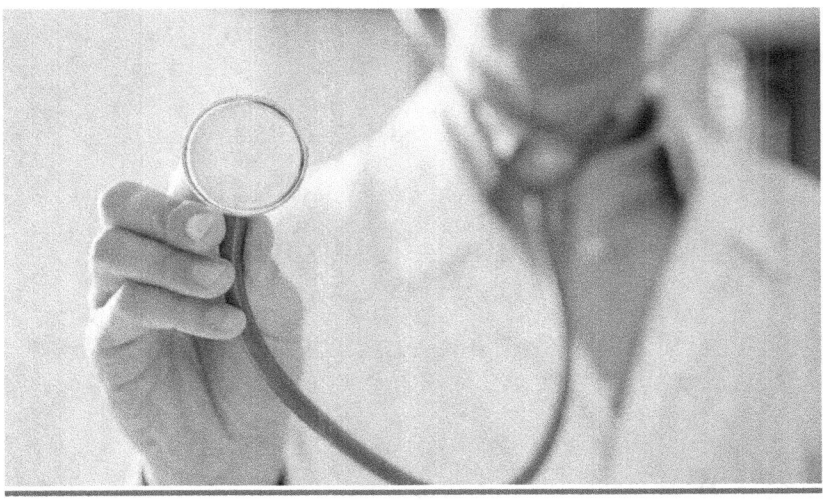

https://www.subscribepage.com/autoimmune

Table Of Contents

Introduction

Chapter 1 – Introduction to the Ultimate Guide on Juicing

Chapter 2 – Juicing 101

Chapter 3 – What Nutrients Are in Fruits and Vegetables

Chapter 4 – Choosing the Right Juicer for You

Chapter 5 – Creating Your Own Juicing Station

Chapter 6 – Detoxing the Body through Juice Cleansing

Chapter 7 – The Best Juice and Smoothie Recipes for Your Various Needs

Chapter 8 – Enhancing Your Juice Cleansing Experience

Chapter 9 – Ending Your Juice Cleanse the Right Way

Conclusion

Resources Page

Claim your FREE Audiobook Now

Introduction

This book contains valuable information about the proper way of practicing juicing as a means of improving one's health and appearance.

Extracting the juice from fresh fruits and vegetables has long been recognized as an effective strategy for losing weight, fighting off diseases, and attaining longevity.

Despite its long history, many people still have the wrong assumptions about this health improvement strategy. There are also some who make juicing seem more complicated than it really is.

Don't miss out on the benefits of juicing just because of these reasons.

To address these issues surrounding juicing, this book is written to serve as an ultimate guide for both beginners and juicing enthusiasts. The topics covered here include:

- the potential benefits and risks associated with juicing;
- the nutritional value of various fruits and vegetables that may be juiced;
- the right way to select juicing equipment and supplies;

- applying juice cleansing as an effective detox technique for the body;

- dozens of juice and smoothie recipes that you can prepare yourself;

- ways to make juicing a fun and rewarding experience for you; and

- breaking a juice fast in the proper way.

Read carefully each chapter, and discover for yourself the secrets of the ultimate juicing formula.

Thanks for buying this book, I hope you enjoy it!

Chapter 1 – Introduction to the Ultimate Guide on Juicing

Juice cleansing, juice fasting, or juicing—you might be hearing a lot about this new fasting trend from fitness experts and health enthusiasts. The thing is, juicing is not exactly a recent trend or a modern invention.

For many generations now, various cultures from different parts of the world have been drinking juices as prevention and remedy. However, despite its long history, juicing has only gone mainstream for the past few years.

Why? If it is so effective, how did it not gain popularity earlier than it did?

The Common Issues Surrounding Juice Cleansing

There are five major factors that have contributed to the current status of juicing as an effective health and weight loss strategy.

1. *Insufficient Information about the Benefits and Risks of Juice Cleansing*

   Many people understandably express their hesitation in adapting juicing as a fasting technique.

   For some, the benefits may seem too good to be true. They simply refuse to believe that fruit and vegetable juices are enough to prevent serious illnesses, and heal them of their injuries and diseases.

Others think that juicing would just be like any other diet fad that have risen and fallen out of popularity through the years. Those people had placed their hopes on strategies that ultimately failed to deliver their expectations.

There are also some people who listen to rumors about the supposed risks of juicing—many of which are not backed by solid research. As such, they give in to their fears rather than consulting those who are better informed about this topic.

2. *A Wide Selection of Fruits and Vegetables to Choose From*

Having a lot of options is a double-edged sword. On one hand, there would be something for everyone. However, choice overload can lead to indecision, and ultimately, inaction.

The same principle applies to the ingredients that may be used for juices and smoothies. You may use only your favorites, but there is no assurance that those would be enough to provide all the nutrients that your body needs.

The decision-making process involved in this is not as straightforward as you might expect. You have to assess your current health condition, and match your requirements against the nutritional value of fruits and vegetables. Even then, there would still be many options to choose from.

It is no wonder that many people feel overwhelmed by just the thought of preparing the perfect juices and smoothies for them.

3. *Uncertainty about the Right Juicing Equipment and Supplies*

There is no single perfect juicer for everyone in the market today. At the end of the day, the right juicer for you would depend on the ingredients, and your personal preferences.

Furthermore, the problems brought about by choice overload may be present in this case as well. A quick search on the web would show you the numerous options that would fit both your requirements and budget. The confusion extends further to the tools and supplies that you may use to supplement your juicer.

Many beginners find the selection process to be daunting. Even some experienced practitioners feel undecided when faced with so many great options to choose from. After all, these are investments that would significantly influence your success at juice cleansing.

4. *Assumptions about Detoxifying the Body Through Juicing*

Due to the lack or lessened intake of solid foods during a juice cleanse, many people assume that their bodies would feel less energized, and that their minds would be hindered from making sound judgment.

Studies show that these negative side-effects do occur for some people, but they are not temporary afflictions. Moreover, the same could be said for other methods of fasting and diet fads.

Despite these and the numerous cleansing benefits of juicing, many people still feel discouraged to try out this strategy.

5. *Complicated Juice and Smoothie Recipes*

A good recipe does not have to include every color of fruits and vegetables in order for it be effective. Some experts at juicing seem to think otherwise, however.

As such, many would-be practitioners find themselves scratching their heads at the overly complicated recipes that are featured in many juicing recipe books.

Furthermore, some ingredients are hard to source, or even unavailable in the local area. Without providing information about alternative ingredients, some people might end up feeling that juicing is not a good fit for them.

6. *Worries and Fears about What to Do Before, During and After a Juice Cleanse*

   Many books only discuss the way to start juicing, or the various recipes that you may try. Only a few resources are available to enlighten you about the entire process that your body would have to go through.

   Some people use this as their basis for claiming that juice cleansing does not work, or that it actually causes harm to the body. What they have failed to notice is that they had skipped some necessary steps to ensure the effectiveness of juice cleansing.

   This book aims to cover these seven factors, thereby addressing all the possible concerns that beginners might have about juicing.

   Those who are currently in the middle of juice fasting may also benefit greatly from this book. There are times when questions only arise when you have begun making changes in your diet and lifestyle.

   Separating the Myths from the Facts

   To achieve such goals, this book is going to explain the essentials of juicing in the simplest terms possible. Through a careful review of the current juicing trends and practices, the author commits to shed light on the following truths about juicing:

- *Benefits and Risks of Juicing*

  Discover the numerous benefits of juicing while learning also the various risks that the method entails.

  Diving into juice cleansing without considering both may only be a time-waster; Doing so may also be harmful to your health and general wellbeing.

  This section of the book condenses the various studies conducted on juicing in order to start off your journey with the right expectations.

- *Nutritional Values of Various Fruits and Vegetables*

  Save yourself from having to research the nutrients contained by your favorite fruits and vegetables.

  For an even better approach, consider adding the top 10 fruits and top 10 vegetables in terms of nutritional content into your juices and smoothies. Find out their respective health benefits as well in order to better determine the best combinations that would work for you.

- *Important Features of Your Juicing Station*

Learn the right way to assess the compatibility of a juicer, as well as various juicing tools, supplies, and boosters, with your health condition and dietary requirements.

You might be tempted to go for the most expensive model, tools, and supplies, thinking that it would be a wise investment in the future. However, the best juicing station for you does not have to be most advanced model there is, at the moment.

Rather than the cost, focus on the features and implements that would help you achieve your fitness goals. Assure yourself that you have made the right decision by going through the guide questions enumerated in this book. Consider your responses as your guide in finding the ideal juicer for you.

- *Effective Techniques to Cleanse the Body Through Juicing*

  Detoxifying the body through juices and smoothies requires a lot of preparation and careful research. Find out everything you need to know about this process before jumping into it.

  Through this, you will gain a better appreciation of juicing as a way to lose weight, increase your energy, and improve the performance of your brain. Ultimately, these benefits would enable you to enjoy a healthier and longer life, especially when you decide to regularly engage in juice fasts.

- *Simple Juice and Smoothie Recipes That Work*

    You do not have to be an expert in the kitchen to make juices and smoothies that are highly beneficial for your body.

    Every recipe in this book indicates the health benefits that you may expect from each. Find out the recipes that will help you achieve specific goals that you may have, such as losing the excess fat in your belly, and obtaining younger-looking skin.

    With the right juice and smoothie recipes, you may improve your appearance and health without having to subject yourself to exhausting workout routines every single day.

- *Easy Strategies to Apply Before, During, and After a Juice Cleanse*

    Dispel your worries and doubts about the process of juice cleansing by learning the strategies that you could follow during various stages of a juice fast.

    Discover the proper way to begin cleansing your body. Then, keep in mind the guidelines that would enhance your experience and the benefits that you can gain from a juice cleanse.

Finally, learn how you can effectively transition from the cleansing phase to a sustainable approach towards a healthier diet and lifestyle.

Overcome your fears, hesitations, and insecurities related to juice cleansing by listening to the pieces of advice given in every chapter of this book.

Take a step closer to the future that you dream to have by making juices as your go-to strategy for weight loss and health improvement.

<u>Through this ultimate guide on juicing, you may start this journey today, the right way.</u>

Chapter 2 – Juicing 101

Before, juices and smoothies are simply part of the menu in restaurants and cafes. Nowadays, you can find dedicated juice bars and smoothie kiosks in malls, parks, gyms, and even in some hospitals.

This growing popularity comes with its own benefits and caveats for consumers, in general. On one hand, you would have plenty of options to choose from—some shops even offer juices and smoothies that are customized according to your preferences. However, the hype surrounding these beverages allows these shops to get away with their high—sometimes unreasonable—prices.

Fortunately, you do not have to be highly skilled in the kitchen to make your own juices and smoothies. With the right equipment, a couple of recipes to start, and a bit of your time, juicing can be as easy as pushing a button or two.

Before delving deeper into the science and art of juicing, you must understand first the basics. Here are the answers to the questions that you might have in mind right now.

- *Are juices and smoothies just the same thing?*

Though both juices and smoothies contain concentrated amounts of vitamins, minerals, and anti-oxidants, these beverages differ from one another mainly in terms of:

- *Ingredients You May Use*

There are certain fruits and vegetables that simply cannot be juiced. Their normal water content is insufficient for machines to successfully extract. Here is a list of the produce that do not work well with standard juicing equipment:

Avocado

Processing an avocado directly into a juicer would only cause your equipment to jam. Rather than avocado juice, most people create dips or smoothies out of avocados instead.

There is a way to include avocado into your juice, however. Simply break down avocado chunks in a blender until the texture has become smooth. Add that into your juice, and stir well.

Expect your beverage to become thick and creamy, though due to the natural texture of blended avocado.

Banana

Similar to avocados, bananas may cause problems to your juicer if you choose to extract liquids out of them.

You may incorporate bananas into your juice by blending them together. Just pour a cup of your preferred juice into a blender, throw in a half banana that has been sliced into chunks, and then blend until the texture becomes smooth.

The result would be more similar to a smoothie rather than a juice. If you prefer something less thick, simply increase the ratio of your juice compared to the banana chunks.

Rhubarb

Though rhubarb leaves are not fit for human consumption, the plant's stalks can be eaten as jams or pie filling.

Unfortunately, the same cannot be said for juices. You would have to extract liquid from several rhubarb stalks to produce a single glass of juice.

As such, the level of toxicity of rhubarb juice far exceeds those contained in rhubarb stalks. Drinking this would cause irritation in the stomach, and certain kidney problems in the long run.

Nuts, grains, and seeds

If you are determined to include them into your juices, you may finely chop them instead, and use that as toppings for your juice. Doing so would provide a nice protein boost to your beverage.

Popular choices include cashew nuts, almonds, quinoa, and chia seeds.

Preparation Method

Homemade juices can be prepared by manual or automatic means. Either way, juicing involves the separation of the liquid parts of a fruit or vegetable from the pulps and fibers.

Manual juicing can be done mostly on citrus fruits, such as oranges and lemons. To do this, all you have to do is squeeze the juice out of the fruits using your own hands.

However, this method is not possible for harder fruits and vegetables, like apple and carrots. For such produce, you would have to rely on a juice extractor. There are various types to choose from, as you would learn later in this book.

Smoothies, on the other hand, require the use of high-powered blenders or food processors. Other than fruit and vegetables, you would also have to add liquid into the mixture. Common choices of liquids include milk, broth, and even self-prepared fresh juices, too.

Texture of the Beverage Itself

Juice is essentially just the water content of a certain fruit or vegetable. Though the exact output that you may expect varies depending on the produce that you have juiced, most juices are thin and fluid.

Smoothies are the exact opposite of that, however. Due to the higher fiber and pulp content, these beverages tend to be thick and rich.

The differences between juices and smoothies also have implications on the functions and benefits that you can expect from each beverage.

Many people drink juice for cleansing and detoxing the body. Some health experts have even designed fasting techniques that are based on various types of juices.

In comparison, many fitness gurus consider smoothies as excellent meal replacements. With the addition of proteins and vegetables, smoothies may have all the essential nutrients that your body needs.

Some meal plans also incorporate smoothies as healthy alternatives to foods and beverages that are eaten as snacks. Studies show that smoothies can make people feel full for a longer period of time compared to common snacks, such as a handful of nuts and a cup of coffee.

Is juicing just another contemporary fad?

Not at all!

Evidence shows that juice cleansing is neither a modern practice nor an ephemeral concept.

The first records go as far back as the ancient human history. The Dead Sea Scrolls contain the life and practices of the Essenes—an Israelite tribe that existed from the 2nd century BCE up to 69 CE.

One of the accounts described in that document revealed that the Essenes mashed pomegranates and figs together to extract the supposed strengthening juice from the said fruits.

Recent scientific research studies on the health benefits of pomegranate and figs substantiate the wisdom behind this ancient practice.

Without the aid of modern technology, how did the Essenes, and other early humans, recognize the remarkable healing potential of extracts from fruits and vegetables?

The answer is quite simple.

Basically, juicing makes it easier for the body to absorb the nutrients naturally contained by fruits and vegetables. Medical experts of the olden days had already identified the various effects of different types of produce on the body. From there, it was only reasonable for them to associate juices with the benefits of the fruits or vegetables from which they have been derived.

Over the years, juicing experts have discovered various combinations that produce specific benefits for the body. As such, this growing number of positive effects sustain the popularity of juice cleansing in this modern age.

What are the benefits of drinking juices?

Juices promote the immediate absorption of nutrients by your body without having to go through extensive digestion. The effects of juices on your health vary depending on the fruits and vegetables that you would use. In general, however, these are the positive effects on your health that you may expect from juices:

Detoxifies and Cleanses the Body

According to the proponents of the juice detox and cleansing diet, this method has long been used by some people as means of getting rid of the toxins inside the body.

Some people draw the distinction between juice detox and juice cleanse, but the truth is, both concepts revolve around the same ideas about the purifying effects of juices on the body.

Juices help out the organs of the body in two ways. First, they aid in flushing the unwanted and harmful substances and particles out of the body. You would notice this when you experience more frequent urination and bowel movements while in the middle of a juice fast.

During a fast, juices also enable different parts of the body to rest and recover. Since they are easier to be digested, several organs would not have to expend so much energy and effort in breaking down juices to make them absorbable by the body.

You may be able to reap these detoxing and cleansing benefits of juices by drinking extract made from green leafy vegetables, garlic, lemon, carrots, and beets. For more detailed information on this, check out chapter 6 of this book.

Improves the Health of the Digestive System

Looking at the convenient yet unhealthy dietary trends nowadays, it should not come as a surprise that several types of digestive problems are on the rise.

Such issues range from simple bloating and irritable bowel syndrome to more serious cases of stomach ulcers, colitis, and Crohn's disease.

Though these conditions may be caused by other factors, the effect on health and quality of life tend to be similar.

Your body would find it harder to absorb the nutrients that you need to function well.

Drinking juices gives your digestive system a much needed break. Natural fibers found, though essential for good health, tend to impose significant strains on your stomach and intestines. Significantly lessening their quantity in your daily diet would give your digestive system enough time to complete the recovery process.

Aids in Losing Excess Body Weight

In most cases, the body feels hunger not due to the lack of food, but rather due to the lack of essential nutrients. Normally, this would be resolved by giving in to the urge to go snacking or even eating a full meal.

Such a habit increases your calorie intake, which then leads to unnecessary weight gain.

Juices can provide you with the vitamins and minerals that your body is actually craving for. A single glass of juice has a greater nutritional value than your usual snacks.

Furthermore, since there is less digestion involved when it comes to juices, you would be able to feel satiated faster than eating an actual meal.

By drinking fresh juices extracted from various fruits and vegetables, you would gradually notice that you do not have to eat as frequently as you usually do.

Examples of commonly juiced slimming fruits include strawberries, lemon, oranges, mangoes, papaya, and cantaloupe.

Vegetables that speed up weight loss include spinach, collard greens, broccoli, and cabbage.

Makes You Feel More Energized

You might have noticed that you feel lethargic whenever you have eaten a particularly large meal. That is not simply a conditioned behavior that you have learned from when you were a kid.

Studies show that this drop in energy level stems from the fact that your digestive system is working hard in processing the huge amounts of food that you have just consumed. This process requires a lot of energy, thus leaving only a fraction to your other bodily and mental functions.

Juices, on the other hand, do not require much energy to be fully digested and absorbed by your body. By removing the hard fibers and other solid components from fruits and vegetables, most of the hard work involved in the digestive process would be taken care of by your juicer.

Moreover, juices contain large doses of vitamins and minerals that are essential in replenishing your energy levels. For example, having a glass of beet juice before exercising would provide your muscles the oxygen and fuel needed to perform strenuous activities. This would then translate to better physical performance and increased stamina.

Increases Emotional Stability, Mental Clarity, and Memory Capacity

Studies also show that many fruits and vegetables contain nutrients that aid in stabilizing one's mood.

As a result, you may lower your risk of developing various mental and emotional conditions, such as migraines, panic attacks, depression, attention deficit disorders, and various neurodegenerative diseases.

Drinking juices made from fruits and vegetables that are rich in B-vitamins would provide a significant boost to your mental performance, too. Whether it is your critical thinking skills, your creativity, or your capacity to remember things correctly, juices may be able to enhance your overall mental abilities.

To unlock these benefits, focus on consuming juice extracts from the following fruits and vegetables: apricots, oranges, grapefruits, peaches, tomatoes, cauliflower, broccoli, spinach, and asparagus.

Improves the Condition of the Skin

According to dermatologists, acne develops whenever dirt and toxins are clogging up the skin pores. This may originate from the environment, or from within.

You may deal with the environmental factors by following a good skin care regimen. For the internal factors, certain types of juices would enable you to cleanse the toxins out of your body.

With regular consumption, you would be able to notice a significant improvement in the appearance of your skin. Some studies even show that juices can prevent the early development of wrinkles and age spots.

Strengthens the Bones

Even though dairy products are still considered by many people as the primary source of calcium, numerous studies in the recent years indicate that a diet that is packed with fresh fruits and vegetables actually contributes more to the prevention of bone-related diseases, such as osteoporosis and osteopenia.

Researchers have discovered that the high acidic content of dairy products, such as milk and cheese, counters the positive effects they have on human bones.

In comparison, juices made from fruits and vegetables that are rich in calcium tend to be low in acid. As such, they are better at promoting the growth, strengthening, and preventing the degeneration of bones.

Promotes Longevity and Delays the Signs of Aging

Juices are packed with various vitamins, minerals, fatty acids, enzymes, and amino acids, depending on the produce that you have used. As such, you would be able to feel the positive effects of these nutrients on your body, including the anti-aging and health-optimizing properties of fruits and vegetables.

Studies also show that juices contain high levels of antioxidants, which protects the body from cancer-causing free radical molecules.

To help you achieve a longer and healthier life, here are some of the highly recommended fruits that you should juice: apples, blueberries, cherries, pineapple, mangoes, papaya, raspberries, and tomatoes.

Certain vegetables are also more effective than others at keeping you healthy and appearing younger-looking than your actual age. These include bell artichokes, bell peppers, cabbage, carrots, kale, spinach, and sweet potatoes.

Take note that you will not observe these benefits with just one or two servings. You need to undergo at least a three-day juice cleanse to feel the difference in your body and mind.

Are there any risks involved in juicing?

Juicing, like other fasting methods, comes with its own challenges. Though the benefits may outweigh the downsides, the negative aspects of juicing still exist.

Here are some of the potential risks associated with juicing:

- *Formation of Kidney Stones*

Studies show that people who are already experiencing issues in their kidneys would be at risk of developing kidney stones when they drink large amounts of juices regularly.

Even people without existing kidney problems may also end up getting kidney stones if they frequently go beyond the recommended daily serving of juices. Remember, too much of a good thing can still be bad for your health.

- *Probable Exposure to Pathogens*

Produce that are used for juicing must be washed well before being processed in the juicer. Otherwise, the pathogens present on the skin of fruits and vegetables would be transferred into your beverage.

Foregoing the process of washing your produce prior to juicing would also expose you to food-borne illnesses when you peel and slice them. There is a chance that you would get injured while doing so. As a result, pathogens would be able to enter your bloodstream.

This applies to store-bought juices as well. Some sellers are either unaware of the proper food safety practices, or simply indifferent about this aspect of their product. Choose juices that have undergone pasteurization or any similar treatment to avoid experiencing serious health problems due to pathogens.

- *Tooth Decay*

According to dentists, the high sugar content of fruit juices can lead to tooth decay—much like what happens when you eat too many candies. Most fruit juices are also highly acidic, thus contributing to the erosion of teeth enamel.

Studies also indicate that tooth decay due to the consumption of juices results from the lesser need to chew. Even though chewing may seem like a chore sometimes, it is actually a natural and important part of normal functioning of the body. It promotes good blood flow into each tooth, thereby keeping them strong and healthy.

- *pH Imbalance in the Stomach*

    Replacing your usual meals would cause significant changes to the pH levels in your stomach. Depending on how you are consuming them, it may cause either a rise or reduction of the gastric acids.

    Such conditions would then lead to various digestive problems, such as indigestion, ulcers, gut leakage, formation of gallstones, irritable bowel syndrome, and diverticulitis.

- *Stress Contributor*

    If you are drinking juices as a way of fasting, not as a supplement to your meals, then your body would experience periods of starvation. As exhibited by numerous studies on fasting, this would cause significant stress to the body.

    If you are incapable of handling and tolerating elevated levels of stress, then juice cleansing might not be a worthwhile experience for you.

- *Eating Disorders*

Any kind of restrictive diet may contribute to the development of eating disorders and body-image issues. This applies to juicing as well because many people adapt this strategy as a weight loss measure.

Limiting yourself to drinking juices only would not only affect your body, but your mind as well. You would often feel hunger and cravings for food that are not allowed during a juice cleanse. Though that is a natural response of the body, your reaction to such sensations and feelings usually causes the problem.

It may lead you to overeating as a way to compensate for the periods of deprivation that you have experienced. This may then turn into an unhealthy pattern that would eventually cause negative effects on other important aspects of your life.

You may also develop a distorted perception of your body, especially when your expectations from juicing is not aligned with what juicing can actually do for you. As such, you may begin thinking that something is wrong with your body, even though you have no solid basis or reason to believe so.

Given these risks, prior to committing yourself to a juice cleanse, you must consider first every angle to check if this is really something you can and want to do.

Where should you get your juices?

Most people opt for either of these two ways: purchase juices from a health food store, or prepare their own juices at home.

- *Purchasing Juices from Stores*

Buying juices is a practical, low-cost approach to juicing. After all, you would have to invest time, money, and effort to craft your own juices in the kitchen.

However, make sure that you are not sacrificing quality for the sake of convenience. Some stores sell commercially produced juices rather than the fresh variants that are packed with the essential nutrients and antioxidants for your body.

Read the label carefully, and examine the ingredients used for the juice you want to buy. More often than not, commercial juices are high in sugar, artificial colors, and flavorings. Your body does not need that. Such content would only contribute to the toxins in your body that you want to flush out in the first place.

If you are dead set on buying juices, head to your local health food store, and check out the different brands that they offer. These stores tend to support juice producers who might have a better understanding of what the body needs from juices.

There are also some online sellers who takes convenience seriously. You can simply browse through their selections, and order how much juice you would be needing. Your order would then be delivered to your doorstep on the date that you and the seller have agreed upon.

For this option, you would likely have access to the reviews of other buyers, so make some time to read through their comments and suggestions. Given the risks associated with juicing, you should buy juices only from reputable sellers.

- *Preparing Your Own Juices*

Going for the do-it-yourself approach grants you complete control over the quality, nutritional value, and cost of your juices. However, you would have to spend a lot of time learning the basics and planning things out in order to ensure your success at this.

Fortunately, this book shall guide you on mastering the ultimate juicing formula that most juicing enthusiasts follow—from selecting the right juicer for you, to discovering the perfect combination of fruits and vegetables that would satisfy your needs and taste buds, from discovering how juicing detoxifies the body, up to applying various enhancements to your juicing experience.

- *Can juices be stored for later consumption?*

Yes, but only for a limited time. Even when stored in the right conditions, the juice must be consumed within 48 hours after it has been first made. This would ensure that you would still be getting most of the nutrients that the juice originally contained.

Some fruits and vegetables are also not made for extended storage, so you would run the risk of your juice going bad if you decide to keep them for much longer than the suggested shelf-life.

The best way to store juices is by transferring them first in bottles that are specifically designed for juicing. These are usually airtight and made of glass. If you are reusing a juice bottle, then be sure to clean it thoroughly and then let it dry completely before pouring your juice into the bottle. Doing so would prevent the spoilage and contamination of your beverage.

Once you have properly sealed the juice bottle, you can then store it inside the refrigerator. Avoid freezing your juice because this would lessen its nutritional value. Instead, keep it on a chilled condition for an optimal storage environment.

Familiarizing yourself with the basics of juicing is a good start for your journey towards a healthier and more sustainable diet. Your next step is to learn the fruits and vegetables that would get you closer to achieving your personal health goals.

Chapter 3 – What Nutrients Are in Fruits and Vegetables

If you think about it, juices can be considered as natural coffee. Drinking the liquid content of fruits and vegetables the same way bears striking similarities with savoring the extracts from roasted coffee beans whenever you have a cup of coffee.

However, unlike coffee, juices are much more flexible when it comes to flavor and nutritional content. Almost every fruit and vegetable can be juiced, thereby giving you plenty of room to be creative with your drink.

This diversity of choices, however, brings forth its own set of problems. How would you know which fruit or vegetable should go into your juice? After all, you are not just doing this for the sake of getting something to drink.

You have goals for the improvement of your health and appearance in your mind, and you are hoping that juices will help you achieve them.

To guide you in making the right selection, here are the top 20 fruits and top 20 vegetables that are packed with essential vitamins, minerals, and antioxidants for your body.

The Top 20 Fruits for Juicing

- *Apple*
  - Nutritional Value (Serving Size: 100 grams)
    - Calories: 52
    - Water Content: up to 86%
    - Carbohydrates: 13.8 grams
    - Sugar: 10.4 grams
    - Fiber: 2.4 grams
    - Protein: 0.3 gram
    - Fat: 0.2 gram
  - Rich in
    - Catechin
    - Chlorogenic Acid
    - Potassium
    - Quercetin
    - Vitamin C
  - Key Health Benefits

- ☐ Lowers the risk of type-2 diabetes by slowing down and regulating the release of glucose into the bloodstream
- ☐ Promotes weight loss through its naturally sweet taste, which may curb your cravings
- ☐ Reduces the risk of various heart diseases by preventing the buildup of plaque in the blood vessels and lowering the bad cholesterol levels in the blood

- *Apricot*
  - Nutritional Value (Serving Size: 155 grams)
    - Calories: 74
    - Water Content: up to 86%
    - Carbohydrates: 17.2 grams
    - Sugar: 14.3 grams
    - Fiber: 3.1 gram
    - Protein: 2.2 gram
    - Fat: 0.6 gram
  - Rich in
    - ❖ Beta-Carotene
    - ❖ Calcium

- ❖ Lutein
- ❖ Magnesium
- ❖ Potassium
- ❖ Vitamin A
- ❖ Vitamin C
- o Key Health Benefits
- ☐ Protects the eyes from free radical damage and oxidative stress
- ☐ Reduces the likelihood of getting sunburned and forming skin wrinkles
- ☐ Promotes the health of gut bacteria, which are essential for normal digestion

- *Blackberries*
- o Nutritional Value (Serving Size: 100 grams)
- Calories: 62
- Water Content: up to 88%
- Carbohydrates: 13.8 grams
- Fiber: 7.6 grams

- Sugar: 7 grams
- Protein: 2 grams
- Fat: 0.7 gram
- Rich in
  - Calcium
  - Iron
  - Magnesium
  - Manganese
  - Vitamin A
  - Vitamin C
  - Vitamin K
- Key Health Benefits
  - Promotes the formation of collagen, which is essential in healing wounds, and regenerating skin cells
  - Improves the health and efficiency of the digestive system
  - Lowers the risk of osteoporosis and epileptic seizures

- *Blueberries*
  - Nutritional Value (Serving Size: 100 grams)

- Calories: 57
- Water Content: up to 84%
- Carbohydrates: 14.5 grams
- Sugar: 10 grams
- Fiber: 2.4 grams
- Protein: 0.7 gram
- Fat: 0.3 gram
- Rich in
  - Anthocyanins
  - Manganese
  - Myricetin
  - Quercetin
  - Vitamin C
  - Vitamin K1
- Key Health Benefits
  - Promotes a healthy oxygen flow in the brain, thus sustaining the optimal condition of neurons and nerve connections

- Prevents the occurrence of early memory decline among the elderly
- Enhances insulin sensitivity by regulating the release of glucose into the bloodstream after you have eaten a meal

- *Cantaloupe*
  - Nutritional Value (Serving Size: 177 grams)
    - Calories: 60
    - Water Content: up to 90%
    - Carbohydrates: 14.4 grams
    - Sugar: 3.9 grams
    - Fiber: 1.6 grams
    - Protein: 1.5 grams
    - Fat: 0.3 gram
  - Rich in
    - ❖ Beta-Carotene
    - ❖ Calcium
    - ❖ Folate
    - ❖ Magnesium

- ❖ Potassium
- ❖ Vitamin A
- ❖ Vitamin C
- o Key Health Benefits
- ☐ Excellent in fighting off the free radicals that can cause significant damage to the cells
- ☐ Keeps the skin hydrated for a longer period of time
- ☐ Improves the condition of your muscles, especially after exercising the body
- *Cranberries*
- o Nutritional Value (Serving Size: 100 grams)
- Calories: 46
- Water Content: up to 87%
- Carbohydrates: 12.2 grams
- Fiber: 4.6 grams
- Sugar: 4 grams
- Protein: 0.4 gram
- Fat: 0.1 gram

- Rich in
  - Myricetin
  - Peonidin
  - Quercetin
  - Ursolic Acid
  - Vitamin C
  - Vitamin E
  - Vitamin K1
- Key Health Benefits
  - Prevents the likelihood of developing urinary tract infections
  - Reduces the risk of stomach ulcers and stomach cancer
  - Improves the overall health and efficiency of the cardiovascular system

- *Grapefruit*
  - Nutritional Value (Serving Size: 230 grams)
    - Calories: 74
    - Water Content: up to 90%

- Carbohydrates: 18.6 grams
- Sugar: 16.1 grams
- Fiber: 2 grams
- Protein: 1.4 grams
- Fat: 0.2 gram
  - Rich in
    - Calcium
    - Folate
    - Magnesium
    - Potassium
    - Thiamine
    - Vitamin A
    - Vitamin C
  - Key Health Benefits
    - Lowers the risk of kidney stones by flushing the waste materials out of the kidney
    - Effective at controlling the appetite by increasing the time needed for full digestion

- Prevents the onset of diabetes by reducing the likelihood of becoming insulin resistant

- *Grapes*
  - Nutritional Value (Serving Size: 151 grams)
    - Calories: 104
    - Water Content: up to 82%
    - Carbohydrates: 27.3 grams
    - Sugar: 23.4 grams
    - Fiber: 1.4 grams
    - Protein: 1.1 grams
    - Fat: 0.2 gram
  - Rich in
    - Copper
    - Potassium
    - Resveratrol
    - Thiamine
    - Vitamin B6
    - Vitamin C

- ❖ Vitamin K
  - Key Health Benefits
    - Lowers the risk of several chronic health conditions, such as heart diseases, various types of cancer, and diabetes
    - Reduces the likelihood of developing eye cataracts, glaucoma, and macular degeneration
    - Improves mental performance by increasing the attention span, and capacity of memory
- *Lemon*
  - Nutritional Value (Serving Size: 100 grams)
    - Calories: 29
    - Water Content: up to 89%
    - Carbohydrates: 9.3 grams
    - Fiber: 2.8 grams
    - Sugar: 2.5 grams
    - Protein: 1.1 grams
    - Fat: 0.3 gram
  - Rich in
- ❖ Citric Acid

- ❖ Diosmin
- ❖ D-limonene
- ❖ Eriocitrin
- ❖ Hesperidin
- ❖ Potassium
- ❖ Vitamin B6
- ❖ Vitamin C
  - Key Health Benefits
    - Reduces the risk of heart diseases and stroke
    - Prevents the formation of kidney stones
    - Hinders the development of cancer cells in the colon, lungs, mouth, skin, and stomach

- *Mango*
  - Nutritional Value (Serving Size: 165 grams)
    - Calories: 99
    - Water Content: up to 83%
    - Carbohydrates: 24.7 grams

- Sugar: 22.5 grams
- Fiber: 2.6 grams
- Protein: 1.4 grams
- Fat: 0.6 gram
  - Rich in
    - Copper
    - Folate
    - Mangiferin
    - Niacin
    - Potassium
    - Vitamin A
    - Vitamin B6
    - Vitamin C
  - Key Health Benefits
    - Provides a significant boost for the immune system
    - Reduces bad cholesterol, omega-6 fatty acids, and triglycerides, all of which contribute to various heart diseases

- Prevents digestive problems, such as chronic constipation and diarrhea
- *Orange*
  - Nutritional Value (Serving Size: 100 grams)
    - Calories: 47
    - Water Content: up to 87%
    - Carbohydrates: 11.8 grams
    - Sugar: 9.4 grams
    - Fiber: 2.4 grams
    - Protein: 0.9 gram
    - Fat: 0.1 gram
  - Rich in
    - Citric Acid
    - Folate
    - Lycopene
    - Potassium
    - Thiamine
    - Vitamin C

- Key Health Benefits
    - Enhances the effectiveness of the body's defense mechanisms
    - Lowers the triglycerides and bad cholesterol levels in the bloodstream
    - Prevents anemia and the formation of kidney stones
- *Papaya*
  - Nutritional Value (Serving Size: 152 grams)
    - Calories: 30
    - Water Content: up to 88%
    - Carbohydrates: 15 grams
    - Sugar: 6.2 grams
    - Fiber: 3 grams
    - Protein: 1 gram
    - Fat: 0.4 gram
  - Rich in
    - Folate
    - Lycopene

- Potassium
- Vitamin A
- Vitamin C
  - Key Health Benefits
    - Protects the cells from oxidative stress
    - Lowers the risk of developing breast cancer
    - Effective at treating irritable bowel syndrome and constipation

- *Peach*
  - Nutritional Value (Serving Size: 154 grams)
    - Calories: 60
    - Water: up to 89%
    - Carbohydrates: 14.7 grams
    - Sugar: 12.9 grams
    - Fiber: 2.3 grams
    - Protein: 1.4 grams
    - Fat – 0.4 gram
  - Rich in

- ❖ Copper
- ❖ Manganese
- ❖ Niacin
- ❖ Potassium
- ❖ Vitamin A
- ❖ Vitamin C
- ❖ Vitamin E
- ❖ Vitamin K
- o Key Health Benefits
- ☐ Promotes smooth and quick digestions
- ☐ Protects the heart and blood vessels by lowering the cholesterol levels, triglycerides, and blood pressure
- ☐ Prevents the growth, development, and spread of cancer cells across different parts of the body
- *Pear*
- o Nutritional Value (Serving Size: 178 grams)
- Calories: 101
- Water: up to 88%

- Carbohydrates: 27 grams
- Sugar: 8.6 grams
- Fiber: 5.5 grams
- Protein: 0.6 gram
- Fat: 0.3 gram
  - Rich in
    - Copper
    - Polyphenol antioxidants
    - Potassium
    - Vitamin C
    - Vitamin K
  - Key Health Benefits
    - Promotes regular bowel movements thus providing relief from constipation
    - Reduces the risk of type-2 diabetes and several types of heart diseases
    - Contributes to faster but healthier weight loss
- *Pineapple*

- Nutritional Value (Serving Size: 165 grams)
  - Calories: 83
  - Water Content: up to 86%
  - Carbohydrates: 21.6 grams
  - Sugar: 16.3 grams
  - Fiber: 2.3 grams
  - Protein: 0.9 gram
  - Fat: 0.2 gram
- Rich in
  - Folate
  - Magnesium
  - Niacin
  - Potassium
  - Vitamin B6
  - Vitamin C
- Key Health Benefits
  - Fights off oxidative stress through the various antioxidants it contains

- Promotes quick and easy digestion by aiding in the breakdown of protein molecules from the food and drinks you consume
- Boosts the immune system and suppresses inflammation across the body

- *Plum*
  - Nutritional Value (Serving Size: 165 grams)
    - Calories: 76
    - Water Content: up to 87%
    - Carbohydrates: 18.8 grams
    - Sugar: 16.4 grams
    - Fiber: 2.3 grams
    - Protein: 1.2 grams
    - Fat: 0.5 gram
  - Rich in
    - ❖ Copper
    - ❖ Manganese
    - ❖ Potassium
    - ❖ Vitamin A

- ❖ Vitamin C
- ❖ Vitamin K
- o Key Health Benefits
- ☐ Regulates the release of glucose into the bloodstream
- ☐ Prevents high blood pressure and elevated levels of bad cholesterol
- ☐ Reduces inflammation in different parts of the body
- *Raspberry*
- o Nutritional Value (Serving Size: 123 grams)
- Calories: 64
- Water Content: up to 86%
- Carbohydrates: 14.7 grams
- Fiber: 8 gram
- Sugar: 5.4 grams
- Protein: 1.5 grams
- Fat: 0.8 gram
- o Rich in
- ❖ Ellagic Acid

- ❖ Iron
- ❖ Magnesium
- ❖ Potassium
- ❖ Quercetin
- ❖ Vitamin C
- ❖ Vitamin E
- ❖ Vitamin K
  - ○ Key Health Benefits
    - ☐ Reduces the amount of carbohydrates that the body absorbs after digesting a meal
    - ☐ Lowers the risk of various types of cancer, such as breast cancer, liver cancer, and colon cancer
    - ☐ Aids in losing excess body weight
- *Strawberry*
  - ○ Nutritional Value (Serving Size: 100 grams)
    - Calories: 32
    - Water Content: up to 91%
    - Carbohydrates: 7.7 grams

- Sugar: 4.9 grams
- Fiber: 2 grams
- Protein: 0.7 gram
- Fat: 0.3 gram
- Rich in
  - Ellagic Acid
  - Folate
  - Manganese
  - Pelargonidin
  - Potassium
  - Procyanidins
  - Vitamin C
- Key Health Benefits
  - Regulates the release of glucose into the bloodstream after a meal
  - Prevents the development of certain types of cancer, such as breast, cervix, colon, and esophagus
  - Protects the heart from damages caused by free radicals

- *Tomato*
  - Nutritional Value (Serving Size: 100 grams)
    - Calories: 18
    - Water Content: up to 95%
    - Carbohydrates: 3.9 grams
    - Sugar: 2.6 grams
    - Fiber: 1.2 grams
    - Protein: 0.9 gram
    - Fat: 0.2 gram
  - Rich in
    - Beta-Carotene
    - Chlorgenic Acid
    - Folate
    - Lycopene
    - Potassium
    - Vitamin C
    - Vitamin K1
  - Key Health Benefits

- ☐ Decreases the oxidative damage and stress in the bones
- ☐ Prevents the growth of cancer cells in the lungs and prostate
- ☐ Lowers the risk of developing cataracts in the eyes
- *Watermelon*
  - Nutritional Value (Serving Size: 100 grams)
    - Calories: 30
    - Water Content: up to 91%
    - Carbohydrates: 7.6 grams
    - Sugar: 6.2 grams
    - Protein: 0.6 gram
    - Fiber: 0.4 gram
    - Fat: 0.2 gram
  - Rich in
    - ❖ Citrulline
    - ❖ Copper
    - ❖ Lycopene
    - ❖ Potassium

- ❖ Vitamin A
- ❖ Vitamin B5
- ❖ Vitamin C
- o Key Health Benefits
- ☐ Promotes the dilation and relaxation of blood vessels
- ☐ Minimize the likelihood of insulin resistance
- ☐ Reduces soreness of the muscles after performing intense exercises, such as running or swimming

The Top 20 Vegetables for Juicing

- *Asparagus*
- o Nutritional Value (Serving Size: 100 grams)
- Calories: 27
- Water Content: up to 93%
- Carbohydrates: 5.2 grams
- Protein: 2.9 grams
- Fiber: 2.8 grams
- Sugar: 2.5 grams

- Fat: 0.2 gram
- Rich in
  - Folate
  - Phosphorus
  - Potassium
  - Vitamin A
  - Vitamin C
  - Vitamin E
  - Vitamin K
- Key Health Benefits
  - Promotes regular bowel movement, and feeds the good bacteria in the gut
  - Lowers blood pressure, thus preventing health complications, such as hypertension and heart diseases

- *Beetroot*
  - Nutritional Value (Serving Size: 100 grams)
    - Calories: 43
    - Water Content: up to 88%

- Carbohydrates: 9.6 grams
- Sugar: 6.8 grams
- Fiber: 2.8 grams
- Protein: 1.6 grams
- Fat: 0.2 gram
  - Rich in
    - Betanin
    - Folate
    - Manganese
    - Potassium
    - Vitamin C
  - Key Health Benefits
    - Protects the heart and blood vessels from being damaged by high blood pressure.
    - Enhances the capacity of the body to perform intense physical activities, such as cycling and swimming
    - Slows down the development of dementia among older people
- *Bell Pepper*

- Nutritional Value (Serving Size: 100 grams)
  - Calories: 31
  - Water: up to 92%
  - Carbohydrates: 6 grams
  - Sugar: 4.2 grams
  - Fiber: 2.1 grams
  - Protein: 1 gram
  - Fat: 0.3 gram
- Rich in
  - Capsanthin
  - Folate
  - Lutein
  - Potassium
  - Quercetin
  - Vitamin A
  - Vitamin C
  - Vitamin E
  - Vitamin K1

- Key Health Benefits
    - Protects the eye from oxidative damage that may be caused by too much exposure to light.
    - Lowers the risk of macular degeneration and cataracts.
    - Effective in addressing the health complications brought about by iron deficiency
- *Bok Choy*
    - Nutritional Value (Serving Size: 70 grams)
        - Calories: 9
        - Water Content: up to 95%
        - Carbohydrates: 1.5 grams
        - Protein: 1.1 grams
        - Sugar: 0.7 gram
        - Fiber: 0.7 gram
        - Fat: 0.1 gram
    - Rich in
        - Calcium
        - Potassium

- ❖ Selenium
- ❖ Vitamin A
- ❖ Vitamin C
- ❖ Vitamin K
- o Key Health Benefits
- ☐ Boosts the defenses of the immune system
- ☐ Regulates the release of hormones from the thyroid gland, thus reducing the risk of various thyroid-related health conditions, including thyroid cancer and hypothyroidism
- *Broccoli*
- o Nutritional Value (Serving Size: 91 grams)
- Calories: 31
- Water Content: up to 89%
- Carbohydrates: 6 grams
- Protein: 2.5 grams
- Fiber: 2.4 grams
- Sugars: 1.5 grams
- Fat: 0.4 gram

- Rich in
  - Carotenoids
  - Folate
  - Kaempferol
  - Potassium
  - Quercetin
  - Manganese
  - Sulforaphane
  - Vitamin C
  - Vitamin K1
- Key Health Benefits
  - Lessens the risk of developing cancer cells in the breasts, prostate, lungs, stomach, and colon.
  - Reduces bad cholesterol in the blood
  - Prevents macular degeneration and other age-related eye conditions

- *Cabbage*
  - Nutritional Value (Serving Size: 150 grams)

- Calories: 35
- Water Content: up to 93%
- Carbohydrates: 8.3 grams
- Sugar: 4.2 grams
- Fiber: 2.9 grams
- Protein: 1.9 grams
- Fat: 0.1 gram
  - Rich in
    - Calcium
    - Potassium
    - Magnesium
    - Vitamin C
    - Vitamin K
  - Key Health Benefits
    - Suppresses inflammations in the joints, heart, and intestines
    - Reduces the risk of lunch cancer

- Protects the heart from being damaged by high blood pressure and bad cholesterol

- *Carrot*
  - Nutritional Value (Serving Size: 100 grams)
    - Calories: 41
    - Water Content: up to 88%
    - Carbohydrates: 9.6 grams
    - Sugar: 4.7 grams
    - Fiber: 2.8 grams
    - Protein: 0.9 gram
    - Fat: 0.2 gram
  - Rich in
    - ❖ Beta-carotene
    - ❖ Biotin
    - ❖ Lutein
    - ❖ Lycopene
    - ❖ Potassium
    - ❖ Vitamin A

- ❖ Vitamin B6
- ❖ Vitamin K1
- Key Health Benefits
  - Lowers the risk of stomach cancer, colon cancer, and prostate cancer
  - Reduces the level of bad cholesterol in the blood
  - Improves the quality of vision and general eye health
- *Celery*
  - Nutritional Value (Serving Size: 101 grams)
    - Calories: 16
    - Carbohydrates: 3 grams
    - Fiber: 1.6 grams
    - Sugar: 1.3 grams
    - Protein: 0.7 gram
    - Fat: 0.2 gram
  - Rich in
    - ❖ Calcium
    - ❖ Potassium

- ❖ Magnesium
- ❖ Vitamin A
- ❖ Vitamin K
- o Key Health Benefits
- ☐ Relaxes the arterial tissues thereby increasing the pressure tolerance of blood vessels
- ☐ Reduces inflammation across different parts of the body
- ☐ Minimizes the damaging effects of oxidative stress on cells
- *Cauliflower*
- o Nutritional Value (Serving Size: 107 grams)
- Calories: 27
- Water Content: up to 92%
- Carbohydrates: 5.3 grams
- Fiber: 2.1 grams
- Protein: 2.1 grams
- Sugar: 2 grams
- Fat: 0.3 grams
- o Rich in

- ❖ Folate
- ❖ Manganese
- ❖ Pantothenic Acid
- ❖ Phosphorus
- ❖ Potassium
- ❖ Vitamin B6
- ❖ Vitamin C
- ❖ Vitamin K
- Key Health Benefits
- ☐ Protects the digestive system from inflammation and constipation
- ☐ Reduces the risk of several chronic health conditions, such as cancer and various types of heart diseases
- ☐ Promotes weight loss by slowing down the digestion process
- *Cucumber*
- Nutritional Value (Serving Size: 104 grams)
- Calories: 16
- Water Content: up to 95%

- Carbohydrates: 3.8 grams
- Sugars: 1.7 grams
- Protein: 0.7 gram
- Fiber: 0.5 gram
- Fat: 0.1 gram
- Rich in
  - Calcium
  - Magnesium
  - Potassium
  - Vitamin A
  - Vitamin C
  - Vitamin K
- Key Health Benefits
  - Prevents the buildup of harmful free radical molecules in the body
  - Reduces the risk of diabetes by lowering the level of blood sugar
  - Keeps the body well hydrated

- *Onion*
  - Nutritional Value (Serving Size: 100 grams)
    - Calories: 40
    - Water Content: up to 89%
    - Carbohydrates: 9.3 grams
    - Sugar: 4.2 grams
    - Fiber: 1.7 grams
    - Protein: 1.1 grams
    - Fat: 0.1 gram
  - Rich in
    - Anthocyanins
    - Quercetin
    - Folate
    - Sulfides
    - Potassium
    - Vitamin B6
    - Vitamin C

- Key Health Benefits
  - Prevents the onset of type-1 and type-2 diabetes
  - Maintains optimal bone health

- *Potato*
  - Nutritional Value (Serving Size: 100 grams)
    - Calories: 87
    - Water Content: up to 80%
    - Carbohydrates: 20.1 grams
    - Protein: 1.9 grams
    - Fiber: 1.8 grams
    - Sugar: 0.9 gram
    - Fat: 0.1 gram
  - Rich in
    - Catechin
    - Folate
    - Lutein
    - Potassium

- Vitamin B6
- Vitamin C
- Key Health Benefits
  - Protects the heart from damages caused by high blood pressure
  - Effective in suppressing the appetite
- *Pumpkin*
  - Nutritional Value (Serving Size: 116 grams)
    - Calories: 30
    - Water Content: up to 91%
    - Carbohydrates: 8 grams
    - Protein: 1.2 grams
    - Fiber: 0.6 grams
    - Fat: 0.1 gram
  - Rich in
    - Copper
    - Manganese
    - Potassium

- Vitamin C
- Vitamin E
- Vitamin K
  - Key Health Benefits
    - Boosts the effectiveness of the immune system
    - Slows down the development of age-related eye conditions
    - Improves the appearance, texture, and health of skin

- *Radish*
  - Nutritional Value (Serving Size: 100 grams)
    - Calories: 16
    - Water Content: up to 95%
    - Carbohydrates: 3.4 grams
    - Sugar: 1.9 grams
    - Fiber: 1.6 grams
    - Protein: 0.7 gram
    - Fat: 0.1 gram
  - Rich in

- ❖ Calcium
- ❖ Potassium
- ❖ Magnesium
- ❖ Vitamin C
- o Key Health Benefits
- ☐ Protects the digestive system from harmful microbes and toxins
- ☐ Prevents the uncontrollable growth of fungi in different part of the body
- ☐ Reduces the risk of developing cancer cells

- *Red Leaf Lettuce*
- o Nutritional Value (Serving Size: 100 grams)
  - Calories: 16
  - Water Content: up to 96%
  - Carbohydrates: 2.3 grams
  - Protein: 1.3 gram
  - Fiber: 0.9 gram

- Sugar: 0.5 gram
- Fat: 0.2 gram
  - Rich in
    - Calcium
    - Potassium
    - Vitamin A
    - Vitamin K
  - Key Health Benefits
    - Effective in keeping the body hydrated
    - Protects the cells from being damaged by free radicals
    - Improves the health and general condition of the eyes

- *Spinach*
  - Nutritional Value (Serving Size: 100 grams)
    - Calories: 23
    - Water Content: up to 91%
    - Carbohydrates: 3.6 grams
    - Protein: 2.9 grams

- Fiber: 2.2 grams
- Sugar: 0.4 gram
- Fat: 0.4 gram
  - Rich in
    - Calcium
    - Folic Acid
    - Iron
    - Vitamin A
    - Vitamin C
    - Vitamin K1
  - Key Health Benefits
    - Slows down the development of the signs of aging
    - Reduces the risk of certain chronic illnesses, such as cancer, cardiovascular diseases, and diabetes
    - Protects the eyes from being damaged by too much exposure to light
- *Sweet Potato*
  - Nutritional Value (Serving Size: 100 grams)

- Calories: 86
- Water Content: up to 77%
- Carbohydrates: 20.1 grams
- Sugar: 4.2 grams
- Fiber: 3 grams
- Protein: 1.6 grams
- Fat: 0.1 gram
  - Rich in
    - Beta-Carotene
    - Manganese
    - Potassium
    - Pro-Vitamin A
    - Vitamin B6
    - Vitamin C
    - Vitamin E
  - Key Health Benefits
    - Protects the eye from damages caused by Vitamin A deficiency

- ☐ Regulates the secretion of insulin into the bloodstream
- ☐ Reduces the risk for cancers of the kidney, breast, and stomach

- *Swiss Chard*

  Nutritional Value (Serving Size: 100 grams)

  - Calories: 19
  - Water Content: up to 93%
  - Carbohydrates: 3.7 grams
  - Protein: 1.8 grams
  - Fiber: 1.6 grams
  - Sugar: 1.1 grams
  - Fat: 0.2 gram

  o Rich in

  ❖ Copper
  ❖ Magnesium
  ❖ Potassium
  ❖ Vitamin A
  ❖ Vitamin C

- ❖ Vitamin K
  - o Key Health Benefits
    - ☐ Lowers the risk of pancreatic cancer and lung cancer
    - ☐ Aids in healthy but quick weight loss
    - ☐ Promotes healthy bones and proper blood clotting
- *Watercress*
  - o Nutritional Value (Serving Size: 100 grams)
    - Calories: 11
    - Water Content: up to 95%
    - Protein: 2.3 grams
    - Carbohydrates: 1.3 grams
    - Fiber: 0.5 gram
    - Sugar: 0.2 gram
    - Fat: 0.1 gram
  - o Rich in
- ❖ Calcium
- ❖ Manganese
- ❖ Vitamin A

- ❖ Vitamin C
- ❖ Vitamin K
- o Key Health Benefits
- ☐ Lowers the risk of several chronic illnesses, such as cancer and diabetes
- ☐ Reduces the likelihood of strokes, hypertension, and heart attacks
- ☐ Promotes the health of bone tissues
- *Zucchini*
- o Nutritional Value (Serving Size: 223 grams)
- ▪ Calories: 17
- ▪ Water Content: up to 95%
- ▪ Carbohydrates: 3 grams
- ▪ Sugar: 1 gram
- ▪ Fiber: 1 gram
- ▪ Protein: 1 gram
- ▪ Fat: 0.1 gram
- o Rich in

- ❖ Folate
- ❖ Magnesium
- ❖ Manganese
- ❖ Potassium
- ❖ Vitamin A
- ❖ Vitamin B6
- ❖ Vitamin C
- ❖ Vitamin K
- o Key Health Benefits
- ☐ Aids in quick and healthy digestion
- ☐ Lowers the risk of developing type-2 diabetes
- ☐ Protects the heart from the effects of elevated levels of bad cholesterol and high blood pressure

Chapter 4 – Choosing the Right Juicer for You

Before going into the details about selecting the perfect juicer for you, you should get a solid understanding first of what you may expect from a juicer.

In general, a juicer is a specialized device used to extract the liquid content from fruits and vegetables. It may be operated by hand, or by electronic controllers. They are not synonymous with blenders, however.

The main functions of each equipment differ from one another, thus producing distinct results. Juicers are designed to separate the solid parts—like the pulp and rind—from the juice itself.

On the other hand, blenders grind together the ingredients into bits. You would have to manually strain out the pulps, in case you do not want them in your beverage.

The differences between the expected outputs from each machine go deeper than the appearance and texture of the beverage. Processing produce through a juicer or a blender would determine the amount of soluble and insoluble fibers that you may gain from fruits and vegetables.

In case you are not familiar with these terms, here is a quick rundown of each type of fiber.

Soluble Fibers

The water in your gut dissolves these fibers to form a thick, gel-like substance that helps you:

- *Better manage your weight and cholesterol levels*

    The gel prevents the absorption of most fats from the food you eat. As a result, you would be able to lose weight quicker, and reduce your risk of developing heart diseases.

- *Regulate the level of glucose in your blood*

    Aside from fats, soluble fibers also slow down the digestion of carbohydrates, thus enabling your body to exert more control over the release of glucose into the bloodstream.

- *Ensure the health and optimal count of good bacteria in your gut*

    Dissolved soluble fibers ferment in the colon. When they do, the resulting substance would feed the good intestinal bacteria. These bacteria serve critical roles in the effectiveness and efficiency of your digestive system.

Insoluble Fibers

This type of fiber cannot be broken down by water. As such, they remain mostly intact after passing through the stomach and intestines.

Though you cannot absorb them per se, insoluble fibers can aid you by:

- *Speeding up the movement of wastes in the intestines*

    Insoluble fibers absorb liquids and other substances in your guts to quicken the formation of stool. As a result, this can help you prevent the development of gastrointestinal blockages, and constipation.

- *Lowering the risk of getting serious colon-related diseases*

    Since your bowel movements would become regular, you can lower your risk of developing hemorrhoids and cancer cells in your colon.

You can get these fibers from the foods you eat, as well as from juices and smoothies. Take note, however, that due to the juicing process, the amount of insoluble fibers that you can get from juices would be significantly lower than what you may expect from blended smoothies.

This does not mean that juices are less healthy than smoothies though. Yes, you are missing out on insoluble fibers left on the pulp of the produce. However, in return, you are getting concentrated amounts of nutrients that could boost not only your digestion, but your overall health condition.

Furthermore, you would still be getting insoluble fibers from the other food that you are going to eat. Excellent sources of these fibers include wholegrains, beans, lentils, nuts, and seeds.

Your diet can, therefore, be significantly improved by eating these foods and drinking juices on a regular basis. To do that, you need to learn how to incorporate juicing into your lifestyle.

The best way to start your path towards that goal is to create juices that satisfy your preferences and health requirements.

Understanding the Basics of Juicers

Preparing your own juice is a relatively straightforward process, especially when you have invested on the right equipment. Learning the different juicing recipes that you can make in your own kitchen, however, requires you to spend some time first in getting to know your options for juicing equipment.

What types of juicers should you consider for your needs? Which features should you look for? How much money would you have to spend for your juicer?

Find out the answers to these questions, as well as other essential bits of information about juicers in the following sections.

Main Types of Juicers

Majority of the juicers available nowadays fall into these categories:

a. *Centrifugal Juicer*

The earlier juicing equipment are designed with centrifugal mechanisms. Models under this category feature a shredder in the form of a spinning basket, and a fine strainer.

When operated, the spinning motion of the basket creates centrifugal force, thus pushing the juice out of the produce. The liquid then goes through the strainer to remove any pulps or fibers that have been forced out as well.

Because spinning introduces oxygen into the juice, expect the juice from centrifugal juicers to be a bit frothy.

Pros:

- Allows more fruits and/or vegetables to be loaded into the feeder per extraction
- Extracts juice in a quick and efficient manner

- More affordable compared to other types of juicers

Cons:

- Produces juices with shorter shelf-life due to the heat-induced oxidation that occurs when the shredder spins
- Requires more frequent stops whenever pulp builds up beyond the capacity of the juicer
- Not capable of extracting most—if not all—of the juices from leafy vegetables

b. *Masticating Juicer (or Single-Gear Juicer)*

The gear of masticating juicers crushes the ingredients to squeeze out the liquid content out of them. A fine strainer is located at the bottom of the gears to keep the pulp and peels from the extract.

The process does not generate heat or friction, so most of the nutrients from the produce are preserved.

Pros:

- Extracts more juice compared to other types of juicers
- Generates less heat due to its low speed, thereby minimizing the oxidation of the juice
- Enables the retention of more nutrients in the extracted juice

- Lengthens the expected shelf-life of the juice for up to 48 hours as long as the juice is kept in chilled condition

Cons:

- More expensive than other types of juicers
- Results to pulpier juices that contain more fibers than expected

c. *Triturating Juicer (or Twin-Gear Juicer)*

Using two interlocking gears, this type of juicer presses the juice out of the produce in a slow manner.

The pulp goes through the middle of the gears where it is shredded and squeezed until almost every drop of juice has been extracted.

Pros:

- Makes juices that have more nutrients in them due to the low-heat process that causes less oxidation
- Enables you to get more juice out of the pulp, thus maximizing your expected yield
- Produces juices that can last up to 72 hours, provided that they are stored right away in the refrigerator

Cons:

- Takes a long time to extract the juice from the pulp
- Requires more time to clean up after use

d. *Hydraulic Press Juicer*

Many juicing enthusiasts consider this type as the best in terms of quality of output and efficiency of the juicing process.

Extraction using this juicer occurs in two phases. First, the fruit or vegetables you are using will be shredded into fine pulp. This would then be collected in a mesh bag placed on a hydraulic press tray.

To start the second phase, you must activate the press through either a button or a lever, depending on the model. This would trigger the application of extreme pressure on the bag, thus extracting every last drop of juice from the pulp.

Pros:

- Doubles the amount of juice extracted compared to the yields produced by centrifugal juicers
- Makes juices that are free from oxidation and foam due to the air-tight extraction process
- Extracts even the nutrient-dense pigments from the pulp, thus creating more nutritious juices

- Lengthens the shelf-life of the juice for as long as 72 hours in the refrigerator

Cons:

- Costs significantly more than the other types of juicers
- Requires more time to create a single batch of juice due to the dual-phase extraction process

Each type comes with its own advantages and disadvantages. Therefore, neither type is completely superior to the other. Selecting the right juicer for you boils down to how well a certain model meets your juicing requirements.

Factors to Evaluate When Choosing a Juicer

Though budget usually sets the limit on the models that would be considered, the specifications and capacities of a particular juicer determine which of the options is worth your money.

As a guide, here is a list of the important factors that you must consider before making a purchase:

- *Size*

Check first the location where you would store and use the juicer. Use that information as a reference when evaluating the dimensions of a juicer.

Bigger models tend to be more stable, especially when in use, but smaller variants can be moved around with relative ease. If you plan to use the juicer only in the kitchen, then feel free to go for big juicers.

Otherwise, consider buying smaller, but more portable juicers that you can carry on your own without much trouble.

- *Horsepower*

A minimum of 0.5 horsepower would ensure that the juicer is not going to burn out while you are using it. This much power is also enough to handle simple juices that beginners usually prepare.

Models with higher horsepower are more appropriate for dedicated juicing enthusiasts, who enjoy experimenting with various ingredients.

- *Speed Settings*

Most people would only need two speed settings to meet their juicing requirements: high and low. The low setting should be enough to handle simple juices, while the high setting must be capable of breaking down tougher ingredients.

Expensive models offer more speed settings, thus enabling the user to customize the extracting process based on the ingredients that will be used.

Check if the juicer also has a dedicated electronic circuitry that ensures stable blade speed while the equipment is being used. Such feature serves as a guarantee on the overall efficiency of the juicer.

- *Reliability*

Branded juicers tend to cost more than lesser-known models. However, with that extra value, you may get more assurance of its quality, and availability of parts and service—just in case you would need them later on.

- *Ease of Use*

Go for a model that does not require a lot of time and effort to set up, operate, and clean.

The more parts a juicer has, the more things you have to assemble and wash. Setting up and disassembling the equipment would also take longer.

For your reference, centrifugal juicers tend to have fewer parts than masticating juicers. Both types, however, include variants that have dishwasher-safe components. Going for such juicers would make the clean-up process quicker and easier.

- *Versatility*

    A good juicer can handle well both delicate and tough ingredients.

    If the settings could not be adjusted accordingly, then you might have trouble in extracting juices from delicate produce, such as leafy greens and fresh herbs.

    Similarly, juicers that are only designed for light to moderate use would not be able to process well harder ingredients, like carrots, beets, and watermelon rinds.

- *Hopper/Feed Tube*

    The larger the hopper is, the larger the chunks of produce you can put in it. Therefore, the size would determine how much cutting and slicing you would have to do before processing the ingredients in the juicer.

    Since you would most likely place the juicer on your kitchen countertop, make sure that the opening of the hopper is still accessible to you, given your own height.

- *Continuous Juicing*

    Most older and cheaper juicers only have a central basket that serves as a receptacle for the pulp. Because pulp accumulates the more juice you extract, you would have to stop operating the juicer when the basket gets filled up.

On the other hand, juicers that push out the pulp into an external container enables the extraction process to continue as long as you have ingredients in the hopper.

- *Output*

Find out how much percentage of juice may be expected from the ingredients that you would put in. Efficient models can extract about 90% of juice from the pulp.

If you want higher outputs, go for juicers that feature an outside container for the extracted juice. Studies show that they leave less pulp compared to variants that only have internal chambers.

- *Noise and Vibration*

Ideally, you should go for juicers that produce a minimal amount of noise and vibration. Some models are so noisy that the user may have to use ear plugs while operating the equipment.

In general, the noisier the juicer is, the stronger the vibrations it produces. This may become a problem later on, especially when the vibrations are strong enough to topple over the juicer itself while it is in use.

Centrifugal juicers and expensive models of masticating juicers tend to be on the quieter side of the spectrum.

To help you evaluate juicers in an objective manner, here is a set of comparison guide questions that covers the essential features and specifications that you should consider.

Making a table out of these guide questions is highly recommended to better keep track of the pros and cons of each model.

You may adopt the following table format for your personal assessment:

Guide Questions	Juicer No. 1	Juicer No. 2	Juicer No. 3
Which of your fitness goals would this particular juicer help you achieve?			
Is the juicer within or above your budget?			
Will the juicer fit in your kitchen or storage area?			
In terms of horsepower/watts, how powerful is the juicer?			
In terms of RPM (revolutions per minute), how much heat can the			

juicer produce?			
How much noise does the juicer generate?			
Does it cause strong vibrations while operational?			
What is the capacity of the cup?			
How large is the hopper?			
Do liquids leak where it is not supposed to while the juicer is in use?			
How much juice is usually left in the pulp after going through the juicer?			
Is it quick and simple to assemble?			
How easy is it to clean?			
What kind of warranty does the seller or manufacturer offer for this juicer?			

Compare at least three models, preferably from different manufacturers. Avoid going beyond five models since you might end up getting confused by your choices.

Getting the Most Value Out of Your Money

Find out the best deals by checking out the offers from at least three different sellers or stores as well. Shop around or browse through the web for promos and discounts that apply to your chosen model.

For your reference, here are some of the most popular juicers that come with high recommendations from experts and juicing enthusiasts alike.

- Centrifugal Juicers
  - Breville Juice Fountain Compact
  - Hamilton Beach Big Mouth Pro
  - Cuisinart Juice Extractor
- Masticating Juicers
  - Hurom Slow Juicer
  - Champion Household Juicer
  - Omega 8006 Nutrition System Juicer
- Triturating Juicers

- Samson Green Power KPE 1304
- Super Angel 5500 Juicer
- Green Star Elite Juice Extractor
  o Hydraulic Press Juicers
- Norwalk Model 280
- Welles Juice Press

Finally, do not purchase a juicer simply because it is on sale. Saving a few extra bucks now is not usually enough to make up for the regrets you might have later on. Take the time to research and compare your options before making a final decision.

By following the guidelines and tips given in this chapter, you would be able to choose the right juicer for you. This step would bring you closer to the goals you are expecting to achieve through juicing. Take the next step forward by making your newly purchased juicer as the highlight of your own juicing station at home.

Chapter 5 – Creating Your Own Juicing Station

Juicing can be easier and faster with the aid of the right tools. Here is a list of the suggested kitchen implements and supplies that should be included in your juicing station:

- Vegetable Brush

    Scrubbing fruits and vegetables while washing them removes traces of pesticides, fertilizers, and chemicals.

    You may also use this for cleaning the mesh and other small parts of your juicer.

- Salad Spinner

    Leafy greens are notoriously hard to clean properly. To ensure that no foreign matter would get into your juice, you would have to wash and wipe dry each leaf.

    Salad spinners make this process easier. All you have to do is place the leafy greens inside the basket, flush them with enough water, and spin them dry by pressing a button or by rotating the crank. You may also use the salad spinner for washing and drying other types of produce that you use for juicing.

- Peeler

This comes in handy when you want to remove the rinds from citrus fruits.

In case you are juicing organic produce, then you also have to peel off the skin before processing them in the juicer. Doing so would minimize the amount of pesticides and other chemicals that might go into your juice.

Ideally, the peeler should be made of stainless steel because they tend to stay sharper for a longer period of time. They are also not susceptible to staining.

- Knife Set

    Though high-quality knives cost a lot, they make good investments in the long run. They would remain sharp and stain-free even with constant use.

    You do not have to buy a full knife set for juicing purposes. For starters, just make sure that you have these types of knives in your juicing station: a paring knife, a medium-sized chef's knife, and a serrated bread knife—a useful tool for slicing through the tough peels of some fruits and vegetables.

- Peeler

    This comes in handy when you want to remove the rinds from citrus fruits.

In case you are juicing organic produce, then you also have to peel off the skin before processing them in the juicer. Doing so would minimize the amount of pesticides and other chemicals that might go into your juice.

Ideally, the peeler should be made of stainless steel because they tend to stay sharper for a longer period of time. They are also not susceptible to staining.

- Cutting Board

You need this for slicing and chopping the produce before processing them in the juicer.

Nowadays, cutting boards come in various sizes, shapes, and materials.

In terms of size, choose one that would be suitable based on the amount and size of produce that you would be using. Large fruits and vegetables, such as watermelon and squash, require bigger-sized cutting boards.

Take into account as well the dimensions of the kitchen counter or table where the cutting board would be placed on while you are using it. Make sure that it would fit within the surface to prevent accidents and inconveniences in the kitchen.

For the material, you may opt to get a classic wooden cutting board. For an eco-friendlier approach, choose a bamboo cutting board instead because bamboos grow faster than trees.

However, if you are on a tight budget, then a simple plastic cutting board would do. Just make sure to replace it regularly to avoid micro-plastics getting into your juice.

- Measuring Cups

These are essential in ensuring complete adherence to the recipe. You may also use a measuring cup to portion the juice that you have extracted.

Measuring cups come in different sizes and materials. Go for stainless steel variants because these do not become stained quickly. Consider getting large measuring bowls as well, in case you are going to juice large amounts of produce.

- Strainer

Juices usually become thick when it contains too much fine pulp in it. Ideally, the juicer should be able to filter these out, but that is not always the case.

Some people can drink the extracted juice as it is. However, if you are not one of those people, then the running the juice through a strainer would make the texture thinner and watery.

Stainless steel strainers work well with any type of produce. You may use plastic ones in case you have a limited budget, but the cost may rack up over time since you would have to replace it more frequently.

Another probable alternative is a nut milk bag. Just make sure that you clean it well in between uses.

- Reusable Juice Containers

Ideally, you should be drinking your juice right after you have made it. This would ensure that the juice would have little to no nutrient loss at all.

However, there may be instances wherein such a practice is not doable. Some people to save time by producing juices in large batches. Others simply cannot do so because their schedules do not allow it.

Whatever the case may be, experts suggest using glass containers for storage purposes. Glass is preferable than plastic or wood because it would not affect the quality or shorten the shelf-life of the juice.

Go for air-tight glass containers, if your budget permits. Otherwise, mason jars can also be great for storing juices, especially if you would be bringing your beverage along with you.

- Reusable Drinking Straws

This one is optional because some containers already come with a straw or a drinking spout.

If you prefer drinking through a straw, however, opt for reusable ones rather than the plastic disposable straws. By doing so, you would keep yourself from contributing to the growing problem regarding non-biodegradable wastes.

There are various options to choose from nowadays. Popular variants include glass straws, metal straws, bamboo straws, and silicone straws. Many sellers offer these along with a carrying pouch and a cleaning brush.

Stock Up Your Station with Juice Boosters

Enhance the benefits of juices to your body by adding these special ingredients into your beverage. Though you are not required to throw them in to your juice every single time you make, it is nice to have these boosters on hand whenever you need a little extra to get you through the day.

- Live Aloe Plant

    Keep an aloe plant nearby so that you can easily add the leaf scrapings into your juice. Picking off a portion or the whole leaf will not kill the plant, as long as you are taking good care of it.

    To incorporate this into your drink, all you have to do is remove the outer covering of the leaf, cut the gel-like substance into tiny bits, and stir those into the extracted juice.

Those who cannot do not want to keep a plant buy bottled aloe juice instead. However, the nutrients contained by store-bought aloe are not as high as what you may expect from fresh, natural aloe.

- Dried Chili Flakes or Bottled Hot Sauce

Studies show that the capsaicin contained in chili peppers are excellent in suppressing and fighting off inflammations in the body. There have also been evidences of the pain-relieving properties of peppers, in general. Some experts also suggest chili peppers as a way of sustaining a healthy metabolism.

You can reap these benefits by simply adding some chili flakes or hot sauce into your drink. A couple of shakes or drops would do for every glass of juice.

- Chia Seeds

Low in calories, but high in nutrients—such qualities make chia seeds a must-have for your juicing station. Just a single tablespoon (about 13 grams) of this would give you extra protein, antioxidants, fibers, and omega-3 fatty acids.

Though chia seeds are tasteless on their own, adding them into the juice would make it absorb the liquid, and gain a bit of flavor. Take note that chia seeds would also make your drink thicker and more filling.

- Flax Seeds

If you are trying to control your cholesterol levels, adding ground flax seeds into your drink would enable you to reduce the bad cholesterol in your bloodstream.

Flax seeds contain a lot of fibers that even a half a teaspoon of this booster would be enough to meet your daily dietary requirement. Mix this in with your juice to ensure a healthy cardiovascular system.

- Maca Powder

This superfood should be a staple for your juicing station. When used in right amounts, maca powder can make you feel more energized, increase your endurance, and sharpen your memory.

Experts suggest adding at least ¼ teaspoon up to ½ teaspoon of maca powder per serving of juice.

- Psyllium Husk Powder

This is another excellent dietary supplement, especially for those who needs to reduce their cholesterol levels.

The great thing about psyllium husk is that it has no distinct flavor of its own. However, it will thicken the water or the juice.

Therefore, make sure not to mix too much of this booster into your beverage. Juicing experts suggest adding only a teaspoon of psyllium husk to reap its benefits without significantly altering the texture of your drink.

- Salt and Pepper

    It is perfectly fine to add some salt and pepper to elevate the flavor of your juice—as long as keep the amount to minimum.

    A sprinkle of Himalayan salt, or a dash of freshly ground pepper into your juice would be enough to enhance the taste of your drink.

- Sparkling Water

    If you want your juice to have a soda-like texture, then add half a cup (about 120 ml) of sparkling water into one serving of juice.

    This would also help in lowering the sugar levels of juices made from certain fruits, like mangoes and pineapples.

- Spirulina

This sea vegetable is an excellent source of iodine. Studies also show that spirulina can enhance the detoxifying properties of juices.

Several health food stores sell this in powdered form, so you can easily keep a stock on hand of this in your kitchen. One teaspoon of spirulina per serving of your juice would be enough to feel the effects of this booster.

- Stevia

This natural sweetener is sold by health stores in the form of powder or liquid drops. Many health experts recommend this as a way to sweeten juices without triggering a sharp spike of glucose in your bloodstream.

Still, it is best to limit yourself to a few shakes or drops of stevia per glass of juice.

- Wheatgrass Powder

Wheatgrass, by itself, has plenty of health benefits. Because of its high water content, you can make juice out of this. However, fresh wheatgrass is not readily accessible for everyone.

Wheatgrass powder, on the other hand, can be found in several major supermarkets and stores. This can also be stored for a much longer period of time than fresh wheatgrass, thus making it easier for you to reap its benefits any time you want.

To boost your juice with this, just stir in a tablespoon (about 8 grams) of wheatgrass. Continue mixing until the powder has been dissolved.

Important Juicing Station Tips for Beginners

Setting up a good juicing station does not end with just learning the recommended tools and juice boosters that you may consider getting for yourself. You must also keep in mind the following tips on how to make juicing easy and fun.

- Feel free to experiment with fruit and vegetable combinations.

  Just like in cooking, personal preferences matter when it comes to juicing. What others find as tasty might not be palatable for you.

  To make juicing a more enjoyable experience for you, try creating your own juice recipes based on your preferred combinations. However, remember to consider your health requirements, and the succeeding tips on recipe creation and ideal produce combinations.

  Take note as well that some of your creations might turn out well, while others might end up as failed attempts at juicing. This is perfectly normal, so don't be disheartened if that were to happen to you. Just keep on exploring to find out which juice combinations would delight your taste buds.

- To make recipe creation easier, just follow the 3:1 rule.

    This rule refers to the ideal ratio of fruits and vegetables to ensure a good balance of nutrients in your juice without ending up with a juice that tastes too bitter or leafy.

    According to juicing experts, the standard recipe formula for juices requires 3 types of vegetables per 1 kind of fruit. Many beginners are also tempted to use as many produce as they want. That can be a mistake because, more often than not, the juice would end up tasting bad.

    Keep things simple by adhering to the 3:1 rule as well the succeeding tips on ingredient combination.

- Combine low-water content produce with high-water content produce.

    You can extract juices from fruits and vegetables with low water content, but expect the yield to be less than what you may expect from high-water content produce. The consistency would also be a bit thicker than the regular watery juices, but not as rich as smoothies.

To increase the yield and make the juice thinner, combine leafy greens, mangoes, and other low-water content produce with cucumbers, celeries, zucchinis, and other produce with higher water content. Again, observe the 3:1 rule while selecting the produce for your juice to create a highly nutritious and tasty drink.

- Thaw out frozen produce before juicing them.

    In general, juices from any frozen fruit or vegetable cannot be extracted through a juicer. You have to thaw that out first before attempting to juice it.

    Frozen produce do not make excellent juices, but they can be used for making smoothies instead. You can either throw them into the blender as they are or after thawing them out.

    For juices, it is still best to stick with fresh fruits and vegetables that are in season and available locally.

- Do not attempt to extract juices from dried fruits or vegetables.

    Dried produce has little to no water content at all. As such, there is nothing for the juicer to extract out of them.

    You might think that soaking them in water for a couple of hours would be a good workaround for this. However, most dried fruits and vegetables are high in salt or sugar. They have also lost a significant amount of their nutrients during the drying process.

Therefore, juices from rehydrated fruits and vegetables would likely have higher salt or sugar content, but lower nutritional value compared to the juices extracted from fresh produce.

- Get the most juice out of leafy greens by wrapping them around harder, round-shaped produce before processing in the juicer.

  Because of the delicate structure and generally lower water content of leafy greens, they do not work well with most juicers.

  Juicing experts suggest wrapping the leaves around coarsely chopped carrots, sweet potatoes, apples, or other harder, round produce. This would enable the equipment to process them without running the risk of jamming the gears or shredder with pulp.

- Prep your produce ahead of time.

  This applies especially to your morning juices, but feel free to do advance prep for your ingredients for other juices as well.

  Ideally, you should only peel, cut, and slice the produce right before juicing them. However, studies show that you can store processed fruits and vegetables in the refrigerator for up to 48 hours.

Just make sure to keep them in air-tight glass containers to prevent the produce from becoming too oxidized and/or dried out while in a chilled environment.

- Peel off the skin from citrus plants, mangoes, and papaya, regardless if they were organically grown.

The skin of most citrus fruits, such as oranges and grapefruits, contains substances that cannot be digested by humans. Studies have also shown that ingestion of these peels would cause digestive upset. Lemons and limes, however, are exempted from this. You may grate their peels to add zest to your juices.

Mango and papaya skins should also not be included when extracting juices from these fruits. Aside from containing irritants that are harmful for the body, these peels can jam up your juicer.

Remember to remove the skins of these fruits before juicing them.

- Save the leaves and stems of produce you use for other dishes, and add them into your juice.

Juice recipes encourage the use of leaves and stems from certain produce, such as strawberries and beets. Those parts are also packed with essential nutrients, and they will not significantly alter the taste of the juice.

Other than the produce you would use for the juice, you may also keep for later use the parts of fruits and vegetables that you do not want to include in your salad or vegetable platter. For example, kale stems and the tops of celery stalks might not look great on a serving plate, but they would be great additions to your juice.

Make sure to store the leaves and stems properly. Glass bowls with air-tight lids are ideal for this purpose. Keep in mind, however, that you can only keep this in the refrigerator for two days at most.

- Avoid adding rhubarb leaves into your juice.

Experts actively discourage the use of rhubarb leaves for juicing—or for human consumption, in general. Not every green and leafy plant parts make excellent ingredients for your juices.

Multiple studies show that the rhubarb leaves contain high levels of oxalic acid—a naturally occurring substance that is toxic to the human body. Furthermore, they taste rather bitter, so adding them to your juice would negatively affect the overall quality of the beverage.

Juicing Trivia #____: You might have heard or read about the toxic properties of carrot greens as well. Dispel your concerns about this because this myth has already been disproven through multiple studies.

Carrot greens are also packed with nutrients, but they do taste herbaceous and bitter—a quality that served as one of the foundations of the said false assumption. They will not harm your body though, so feel free to use them as long as you do not mind a little bitterness to your beverage.

- Remove the hard pits and seeds from particular types of produce before juicing them.

    Hard pits of fruits, such as peaches, mangoes, apricots, and cherries, can cause significant damage to your juicer. Furthermore, some studies show these pits actually contain substances that are toxic to the human body.

    Similarly, seeds from apples and pears have cyanide in them. Even in small amounts, this substance can cause severe irritation for those with sensitive stomachs. Pick out the seeds of these fruits before placing the apple or pear slices into the juicer.

- Alternately juice hard produce with softer produce.

    By doing so, you would prevent putting too much strain on your juicing equipment. This would also allow you to get more liquids out of your produce, especially if you are using a centrifugal juicer.

Good juicing recipes indicate the right order of the produce that would be juiced. In case the juicing recipe you are following does not have such instructions, or if you are creating your own recipe, just go first with soft produce, such as berries and watermelon slices, to warm up the juicer.

Tough and dense produce, such as apples or carrots, should go next into the juicer. Repeat this cycle until you have extracted the juices from all the fruits and vegetables included in the recipe.

- Create a juice-smoothie combo by blending your juice with banana or avocado.

Juices, on their own, can be quite filling and exciting to drink. However, if you are seeking for something more substantial, try combining your juice with richer produce, like banana or avocado.

These fruits do not work well with juicers due to their low water content. They can be mixed with juice by breaking them down first in a blender or food processor. You can use the juice itself as the liquid component of the smoothie, thus creating a juice-smoothie combo.

Aside from being highly nutritious, this combination would introduce a new taste profile to your typical juice. The texture would be more similar with a smoothie than a juice though. If you want something thinner, simply increase the amount of juice, or just add half of the banana or avocado that you should have used for this.

- Use air-tight glass containers when you have to store your juice in the refrigerator.

Juices lose a lot of nutrients when they are exposed to air, heat, or light for too long. To prevent this from happening, store your juice in an air-tight, opaque glass container, and place it inside the refrigerator.

Make sure to fill up the container to the brim to lessen the amount of air that would be trapped inside. Keeping air out of your juice would not only stop discoloration from happening. Studies also show that extended exposure to air triggers the oxidation process, thus turning some types of juices toxic for the human body.

Juicing Trivia ____: Juices from cruciferous vegetables, leafy greens, and melons tend to go bad quicker than other variants. Try to consume such juices within the same day they were made. Otherwise, you might have to throw away the excess rather than risk causing harm to your health.

- Re-use the pulp by composting them, or by using them for cooking other foods.

Though most of the nutrients have already been removed during the extraction process, pulps can still enrich the soil when composted properly. If you are taking care of your garden, you can then use the nutrient-dense soil to promote the healthy growth of your plants there.

If gardening is not one of your hobbies, then you can turn the pulp as a healthy extender for soups, sauces, jams, and more. There are plenty of recipe nowadays that allows the use of pulp in cooking.

Consider applying these tips to get the most out of the fruits and vegetables that you buy for juicing.

- Clean your juicing equipment and tools right after using it.

Though this might seem as an obvious thing to do, there are still people who do not see this as a post-juicing requirement.

Some feel too excited about the juice they have made that they fail to clean up their juicing stations right away. Delaying this would only make things harder later on because the hardened residue from the produce can be quite tough to remove.

- For faster cleanup, use a paper bag or plastic bag to line the pulp basket.

Much like regular trash bins, the basket where the dried up pulp goes may be lined with paper bag or plastic bag. This would save you time when you have to wash up the pulp basket after using the juicer.

Used paper bags may be prone to breakage when wet, but they are the eco-friendlier option between the two. If you are going to use plastic bags, avoid buying new ones just for this purpose. Opt to use the ones that you have gotten while shopping for goods instead.

Following these tips would enable you to accomplish one of the main purposes for creating your own juicing station, which is the full integration of juices into your lifestyle and diet.

Nowadays, juices are not only meant for cleansing, detoxing, or fasting. Several experts agree that juicing can fill in the nutrient gaps created by the vast amounts of processed foods that are readily available for everyone.

Chapter 6 – Detoxing the Body through Juice Cleansing

Various health blogs and magazines promote the concept of detox diets as a way to lose weight, prevent diseases, and several other health benefits. The premise is quite simple: restricting your calorie intake would enable you to get rid of the accumulated toxins in your body.

Given the juices and smoothies have significantly lower calories than standard meals and snacks, many detox diet plans encourage their followers to consume only these beverages during the cleansing period.

Much like juicing, however, detox diet is not an entirely new idea. In fact, there is evidence showing that the ancient Egyptians had practiced detoxification thousands of years ago. The Native Americans, even before the arrival of the colonists, remove toxins from their bodies through purification ceremonies.

In the early part of the 20th century, medical experts had devised several ways to potentially detoxify the body. These methods include enemas, bloodletting, and extended fasting, among others.

Looking at its history, detoxing has always been, and will continue to be a subject of interest pursuit for many people. However, despite its long history, the science supporting many of these detoxification techniques are not as solid as you might expect.

Juice cleansing, a popular detox technique, has exhibited great potential in delivering the expected results from this initiative. In this chapter, you will discover why juices and smoothies make excellent detoxification and fasting tools. You will also learn of the many benefits and risks associated with juice cleansing. All the important things to consider when engaging in a 30-day juice fast can also be found at the end of this chapter.

To start things off the right way, you should understand the basics of toxins, detox, and their respective effects on each other and your body.

- What are toxins?

    There are several pollutants or substances that can cause you harm when your body becomes exposed to them frequently or for long periods of time. Common sources of toxins include:

    o Artificial food additives

    o Antibiotics or hormones used on livestock, such as chickens, cows, and pigs

    o Traces of chemicals on the packaging materials for food

- Pesticides
- Household cleaning chemicals
- Detergents
- Vehicular smoke
- Cigarette smoke
- Illegal drugs

The body absorbs these toxins through various means—ingestion, inhalation, touch, among others. People who consume large amounts of commercially produced foods and beverages are particularly vulnerable towards these toxins.

When the body is left in such a poor state for too long, the risk of developing chronic diseases would become significantly higher. These diseases include different forms of cancer, diabetes, cardiovascular diseases, and neurodegenerative diseases.

- How does the body naturally handle toxins?

Numerous studies show that body is continuously engaged in its own detoxification process. Different body organs are involved for the various types of toxins that enter the body.

- Lungs

The tiny hair-like structures in your lungs called cilia serves as a trap for the toxins that may enter the body whenever you breathe in. Once trapped, your body would try to expel the irritant by coughing.

- Liver

The toxins in the blood are filtered out in the liver. That is why those who abuse alcohol, drugs, and those who eat too much unhealthy foods tend to develop serious liver problems.

- Colon

Once the small intestines are done absorbing the nutrients from the food and drink you have consumed, the wastes would go to the large intestines. The colon would then absorb the remaining water and electrolytes before letting the waste—along with the toxins—be excreted out of your body in the form of a stool.

- Kidney

Blood cells pass through the kidneys to remove the toxins they have accumulated while going around different parts of your body. Upon reaching a certain amount, these toxins would then be expelled from the kidneys as urine.

Therefore, even though the body is continually exposed to toxins, you are naturally equipped with defense mechanisms that can effectively handle these potential dangers—but only up to a certain extent.

- What is a detox?

Detox diets are designed to boost your body's natural defenses. Even though there is no universal way to detox the body, the main purpose of each detox method is constant: to aid the body in getting rid of the toxins from an external source.

Most detox diets claim that their plans would essentially cleanse the body, while others simply aim to reduce the consumption of less nutritious foods. Juice cleansing falls somewhere between the two ends.

Also referred to as a juice fast, this detox method would require you to only consume juices made from fruits and vegetables for a certain period of time.

Due to some criticisms about the insoluble fiber content of juices in general, some variations of juice cleansing allows the incorporation of smoothies into the diet plan. Aside from making you feel fuller and aiding your digestion, this would also give you a boost in proteins, fats, and other vitamins and minerals that are essential for the body.

- How do juices remove toxins from the body?

According to the advocates of juice cleansing, this method works by supporting the internal detox processes of the body. Since you would only be allowed to drink natural juices, refined sugars, processed foods, and caffeine would be eliminated from your daily diet.

Furthermore, juices are packed with vitamins and minerals that can be more easily absorbed by the body. The additional fluid intake would also help in flushing out the bodily wastes and toxins that have accumulated inside.

A juice fast, however, is not simply just drinking a glass of juice in replacement of your usual meals. It actually occurs in three stages—each with its own set of guidelines that must be observed for a successful cleansing of the body.

Phase #1: Preparation

This phase should begin around three to five days prior to your scheduled juice cleanse. During this period, you must gradually remove certain kinds of food from your diet, such as:

- coffee
- alcohol
- anything with refined sugar in it
- dairy products

- meat products
- wheat

As a replacement, increase your consumption of fresh, fruits, vegetables, tea and water. This would enable your body to get ready for the upcoming significant changes during the next phase.

Expect some negative side-effects, however, since your body would essential go through a withdrawal. This especially applies for those who are used to a high-sugar and/or high-caffeine diet. Common side-effects include headaches, restlessness, and fatigue.

On the bright side, the inconvenience and ill feelings you would experience during this phase are less intense compared to what you would have felt if you choose to push through with a juice fast without any preparation at all.

Your body would have more time to get acclimatized to the changes in your diet, thus reducing the severity of the withdrawal symptoms that usually accompany fasting and detox diets.

Phase #2: Cleansing

The actual duration of this phase varies depending on the fasting plan that you are following. Beginners usually do it for only one to three days only, but more experienced juice enthusiasts can go for up to 30 days.

Experts recommend drinking no more than 32 ounces (almost 1 liter) of juice per day. The nutrient count of each serving of juice is usually enough to satisfy your daily nutrient requirement. Therefore, going over the said limit can actually be harmful for your health.

Remember to space out each serving throughout the day. You should vary the produce that you would use for each beverage to diversify the nutrients that you can gain during this period.

Make sure that at least half of your daily juices and/or smoothies are high in green vegetables, too. This would enable you to reap a lot of health benefits while toxins are being flushed out of your body.

Phase #3: Reintegration

After the fasting period is over, you must slowly bring in back more solid foods into your diet. Avoid reverting back to your poor food choices though. Stick to lean proteins, fresh fruits, and vegetables so as to maintain the effects of the juice fast longer.

For more information about this phase, check out chapter 9 of this book.

Benefits of Detoxifying via Juices and Smoothies

Now that you have a deeper background on detox and juice cleansing, you would be able to better understand and appreciate the benefits you may expect from this practice.

Take note that the following effects would not be noticeable right away. Your body must undergo the complete detox process to feel the difference that this would bring to your health and the general quality of your life.

- Weight Loss

Juice cleanses can help you quickly lose weight. This stems from the fact that short-term juice cleanses are effective at getting rid of water weight rather than excess fat stores in the body.

- Productivity

Because you are saving on your energy that is usually allocated for digesting food, you would have more resources to perform other tasks—physical or mental ones.

- Increases Mental Clarity

Juices that are made of folate-rich produce would give your mind a boost. Furthermore, studies show that feelings of hunger can heighten one's focus and mental clarity. As with other fasting techniques, being in a juice fast would increase the frequency and intensity of your hunger pangs.

- Cleanses Your Body

    Juice cleanse helps remove environmental toxins that have accumulated in your body. This method is particularly more effective at this than other detox methods because juices hastens the process of flushing out the toxins right out of your body.

The Various Risks Associated with Detox Diets

Juice cleansing is not an ideal or viable practice for everyone. Studies show that certain groups of people are prone to suffer from the probable negative effects of this detox method, such as

- physical weakness
- acne
- muscle pain
- indigestion
- halitosis
- excessive diarrhea

Given these risks, everyone is encouraged to check with their respective physicians first before engaging in a juice cleanse—even more so the following categories of people:

- Children
- Pregnant or nursing women
- The elderly
- Individuals with type-2 diabetes, cancer, or autoimmune diseases
- People who are suffering from kidney, liver, or gallbladder issues

As with any other type of diet, it is best to consult first with your physician if you are physically capable of handling the difficult aspects and negative side-effects of juice cleanses.

The Makings of the Greatest Detox Juice

Not all detox juices provide the same benefits. As such, there is not exactly a single greatest detox juice that would work for everyone. What experts know is that there are certain types of produce that enhance the benefits that you may expect from detoxifying your body.

To help you better evaluate whether or not a certain recipe would result to the greatest detox juice for you, here are the top 10 fruits and vegetables that are well-known for their cleansing properties. Recipes that feature these produce as ingredients are more likely to be more effective at detoxification than other types of juices.

1. Beets

- Eliminates the toxins that have built up in the liver
- Provides the essential nutrients for the proper functioning of the liver

2. Broccoli

- Fights off toxins that can lead to the growth of cancer cells
- Stimulates the production of helpful enzymes in the body

3. Carrots

- Contributes in flushing out the toxins from the body
- Prevents the growth and development of cancer

4. Garlic

- Stimulates the liver enzymes that act as filters for the toxins that pass through this organ
- Suppresses the growth of tumors in different parts of the body

5. Green Tea Leaves

- Prevent the formation of carcinogens in the body
- Reduce the likelihood of developing tumors
- Enhances the cleansing abilities of the liver

6. Leafy Vegetables (kale, mustard greens, spinach, wheatgrass, etc.)

- Aids in flushing out traces of pesticides and heavy metals in the body
- Suppresses genetic mutation of the cells, which may lead to tumors and cancer

7. Lemons

- Transforms toxins into water soluble materials, thus making them easier to break down and eliminate
- Quickens the process of flushing out the toxins from the body

8. Sesame Seeds

- Protects the liver from being damaged by alcoholic drinks and other chemicals you ingest
- Enhances the detoxifying capabilities of the liver

9. Tomato

- Stops the formation of carcinogens in the body

- Prevents the growth and development of cancer cells in certain areas of the body

10. Watercress

- Flushes out the toxins from the kidney
- Increases the frequency of expelling urine from the body

For recipes that feature these ingredients, check out the next chapter. Evaluate the needs and condition of your body first to determine which of those recipes would be the greatest detox juice for you.

Guidelines and Reminders for a 30-Day Juice Fast

A standard 30-day juice fast is primarily composed of juices made from fresh fruits and vegetables. As its name suggests, it is one of the most intense juicing regimens that you can ever experience. Therefore, you must be fully committed and well prepared before starting this challenge.

The thing is, consuming only juices and water for an entire month can lead to disastrous consequences for your overall wellbeing. Many people report feeling minor side-effects like low energy, and intense hunger pangs, but some experience more severe conditions, such as various types of nutrient deficiencies, digestive problems, and physical fatigue.

At this point, you might be wondering why would even bother with something so difficult and potentially harmful for you? After all, there are shorter versions of juice fasts that even beginners can do without much trouble.

To answer this question, you should consider first the reasons why you are planning to undergo a juice cleanse. Are you doing this to lose weight, and perhaps gain some muscle mass in the process? Or maybe you simply want to refresh your system by flushing out the toxins inside your body?

- Weight Management

If you are doing this to lose weight, then the 30-day juice would address one of the popular criticism against juicing in general. Studies show that short-term juice cleansing would only enable you to lose water weight rather than burn off the excess fat stores in your body. Water weight can easily be regained once you are done with the fast, hence the assumption that juice fasts are not effective weight loss tools.

Such an observation stems from the brief duration of the fast itself. With a 30-day period, however, your body would have enough prep time and cleansing time to actually kick-start the process of lipolysis—or more commonly known as the fat-burning activities that happens when you have successfully limited your calorie intake.

- Health Improvement

    Furthermore, the 30-day fasting period would enable your body to undergo a full reset rather than just a temporary one that you would get from short-term fasts. The extended time for fasting allows the completion of the detox process across different parts of your body. This is simply not possible with a quick 1-day juice fast.

    Given such benefits, it is no wonder that many people have already successfully undergone a 30-day juice fast.

    You might still be worried about the potential consequences of this detox method to your health. Fortunately, you are not required to abide by the strict rule against consuming anything other than juices. In fact, some programs encourage beginners, casual practitioners, or those with more active lifestyles to incorporate smoothies and some solid foods into the fasting plan.

    Given these, the objective of a 30-day juice is not exactly to limit yourself only to juices and water. Rather, it is to replace the parts of your diet that are harmful for your body with healthier choices and practices. This would then enable to a smoother and more successful transition to a better diet and lifestyle.

For your guidance, here are the important points you have to keep in mind when taking on the challenge of a 30-day juice fast:

- As with any kind of juice fast, you must prepare your body for the coming changes. Gradually decrease first your consumption of caffeinated drinks and alcoholic beverages. Then, at least 2 days before the fast itself, avoid eating any type of processed foods.

- Plan ahead the types of juices that you would be making for your scheduled fast. Better yet, plot these your plan into a calendar or journal so that you can easily keep track of what you should be preparing and drinking for each day.

  The next chapter covers several juice and smoothie recipes that you should try making in your juicing station.

- Go for organic fruits and vegetables if they are within your budget and are readily available in the local market. If not, just make sure to thoroughly wash the produce with a specialized cleansing agent that will remove all traces of pesticides and other chemicals from the peel.

- For optimal results, you should aim to create your own beverages during the fast. Doing so would allow you complete control over the contents of the juices that you are going to drink.

- Remember to set at least a 2-hour b2reak between each intake of juice. This would keep your hunger pangs to a minimum. Doing so would also prevent spikes up in your blood sugar level.

- For the last drink of the day however, you should consume it at least 3 hours before going to bed. This would give your digestive system enough time to process and absorb the nutrients in the beverage you have consumed.

- If you are uncertain on which types of juice to plot into your schedule, here is a quick reference guide to get you started:

    o Morning: Fruit-Based Juice/Smoothie

    This would give you enough natural sugars to power you through most of the day. You can easily burn through the additional calories from such beverages since you are keeping your intake of solid foods to a minimum.

    o Lunch: Combination of Vegetable and Fruit Juice

    Follow the 3:1 rule for this juice—3 vegetables and 1 fruit. Such a drink would give you a nice boost of energy and nutrients.

    o Dinner: Vegetable-Based Juice

Give yourself a large helping of vegetables, especially the leafy greens and cruciferous vegetables. Feel free to add lemon your dinner juice to sweeten it up a bit, and balance out its nutritional value.

- Aside from lemon, spices and herbs may be used to make your juices and smoothies more exciting and palatable. They also have their own set of nutrients, thereby boosting the health benefits of your drink. Popular choices include:
  - turmeric
  - cinnamon
  - parsley
  - cilantro
- Drink lukewarm or room-temperature water in between your juices or meals in order to sustain the continual flushing out of wastes and toxins from your body
- In case you getting tired of juices and smoothies, here are some other foods and drinks that you may consume during a juice cleanse:
  - almond milk
  - vegetable broth

- raw vegetable sticks made from carrots, turnips, cucumbers, bell peppers, etc.

- gluten-free vegan meals, such as salads and clear soups

    To keep you from wasting all the efforts you have made so far, eat only these foods if the hunger pangs become too uncomfortable for you to bear. This would prevent your level of blood sugar from fluctuating during the fasting period. When this occurs, you would find it harder to get over the symptoms of withdrawal.

- For better absorption of nutrient, try to drink your juice in a slow, little sips. Some people tend to gulp it down because they do not like the taste and/or texture of the beverage. Avoid doing so because it strains out your digestive system, and may even prevent your body from fully absorbing the

Much like other diet plans and fasting methods, detoxifying the body through juice cleanses comes with its advantages, drawbacks, and risks. You may choose to push through with this if its benefits align with your personal goals, if you can accept the flaws of this concept, and if you would not be put at a serious risk by your decision to do so.

Should you choose to undergo a juice fast, you must learn the various recipes that you can recreate at your juicing station. To help you move forward in your journey towards weight loss and excellent health condition, the next chapter will teach you juice and smoothie recipes that would cater to your specific needs

Chapter 7 – The Best Juice and Smoothie Recipes for Your Various Needs

Everything that you have learned so far in this book has prepared you for applying the ultimate juicing formula within the comforts of your own kitchen.

You have discovered which fruits and vegetables can be juiced, and which ones contain the nutrients that your body requires. Your juicing station is equipped with the best juicer that would enable you to achieve your personal juicing goals. You have also learned the essentials of detoxing the body through juice cleansing.

Now, you must take the next step forward by learning how to prepare your own juices. Here are the suggested juice and smoothie recipes that you should try right away.

Juices for Losing Your Belly Fat

Other diets and products claim to deliver quick results without mentioning that they would be robbing you of important vitamins and minerals in the process. The following recipes for nutrient-packed juices, however, would help you achieve a slimmer waist in no time at all.

- *Carrot-Celery Juice*

- Ingredients
- ✓ 3 baby carrots
- ✓ 2 celery stalks
- Procedure

1. Peel and chop the carrots.
2. Chop the celery, but keep the leaves intact.
3. Place the carrots and celery into the juicer.
4. Extract the juice from the pulp.
5. Pour into your preferred container.
6. Stir or shake well before drinking.

- Expected Yield: 1 cup of juice
- Additional Health Benefits
- ❖ Lowers your cholesterol level
- ❖ Improves your vision
- Nutritional Value
- ☐ Calories: 155
- ☐ Carbohydrates: 40 grams
- ☐ Sugars: 19 grams

- Fiber: 11 grams
- Protein: 4 grams
- Fat: 0.23 grams
- Sodium: 0.20 grams

- *Apple Cinnamon Juice*
  - Ingredients
    - 3 green apples
    - 1 teaspoon ground cinnamon
  - Procedure
    1. Remove the core from the apples, but keep the peel on.
    2. Place the apples into the juicer.
    3. Extract the juice.
    4. Transfer into your favorite container.
    5. Stir in the ground cinnamon.
  - Expected Yield: 1.5 cups of juice
  - Additional Health Benefits
    - Effective in satisfying your cravings for sweet treats

- ❖ Fights off bacterial infections in your body
- Nutritional Value
  - Calories: 136
  - Carbohydrates: 37 grams
  - Sugars: 27 grams
  - Fiber: 6.2 grams
  - Fat: 0.63 grams
  - Protein: 0.09 grams
  - Sodium: 0.003 grams

Extra Juicing Tip: Any variant of apple would do for this recipe, but Granny Smith apples are preferable due to their greater fat-burning capabilities than other types.

- *Orange-Watermelon Juice*
- Ingredients
  - 1 orange
  - 1 slice of watermelon
- Procedure

1. Peel and remove the pith from the orange.
2. Remove the rind from the watermelon.
3. Cut the watermelon into cubes.
4. Place the orange and watermelon cubes into the juicer.
5. Extract the juice from the ingredients.
6. Pour into a glass or bottle.
7. Stir or shake well the juice before drinking.

- Expected Yield: 1.5 cups of juice
- Additional Health Benefits

❖ Reduces water retention thereby lowering the risk of feeling bloated

❖ Excellent at suppressing inflammations in the body

- Nutritional Values

☐ Calories: 110

☐ Carbohydrates: 28 grams

☐ Sugars: 22 grams

☐ Protein: 2.9 grams

☐ Fiber: 2.8 grams

- Fat: 0.48 grams
- Sodium: 0.002 grams

Extra Juicing Tip: Go for a mini watermelon—about the size of a small cantaloupe—if it is available. Its size is perfect for individual consumption.

- *Lemon-Lime Juice*
  - Ingredients
    - 1 lemon
    - 1 lime
    - 1 cup sparkling water
  - Procedure
    1. Divide the lemon and lime into two, but keep their rinds intact.
    2. Place the lemon halves and lime halves into the juicer.
    3. Extract the juice.
    4. Pour the juice into your favorite container.
    5. Add the sparkling water.

6. Stir or shake until the sparkling water is mixed well with the juice.

7. Consume immediately.

- Expected Yield: 1.25 cups of juice

- Additional Health Benefits

❖ Helps in curbing your cravings for fatty foods

❖ Contributes to the elimination of impurities in the liver

- Nutritional Value

☐ Calories: 42

☐ Carbohydrates: 19 grams

☐ Fiber: 7.4 grams

☐ Protein: 1.7 grams

☐ Sugars: 1 gram

☐ Fat: 0.51 grams

☐ Sodium: 0.007 grams

Extra Juicing Tip: Make sure to drink immediately any beverage containing fresh lemon juice. According to studies, lemon loses about 20% of its Vitamin C content after 8 hours of being kept in ambient temperature.

- *Cantaloupe-Garlic Juice*
  - Ingredients
    - ¼ cantaloupe
    - 2 whole garlic cloves
    - 1 sprig fresh baby dill
  - Procedure
    1. Remove the skin of the cantaloupe and garlic.
    2. Place the peeled cantaloupe and garlic into the juicer.
    3. Extract the juice from the said ingredients.
    4. Pour into your preferred glass.
    5. Stir well.
    6. Garnish with dill.
  - Expected Yield: 1 cup of juice
  - Additional Health Benefits
    - Reduces water retention
    - Excellent in making you feel energized for a longer period of time

- Nutritional Value
  - Calories: 86
  - Carbohydrates: 24 grams
  - Sugars: 14 grams
  - Protein: 2.8 grams
  - Fiber: 2.1 grams
  - Fat: 0.57 grams
  - Sodium: 0.03 grams

Juice for Amazing Skin

Each of the recipes below would make your skin glow, and prevent the early appearance of the various signs of aging. You can be assured of these promises because these juices are packed with the essential vitamins and minerals for a healthier, smoother skin.

- Tropical Juice
- Ingredients
  - ✓ 1 small pineapple
  - ✓ 1 mango

- ✓ 1 cucumber
- ✓ ½ lemon
- Procedure

1. Remove the peel of the pineapple before cutting it into chunks.
2. Remove the skin and pit of the mango.
3. Peel off the skin of the cucumber, but keep its seeds.
4. Cut the lemon into thin slices without removing its rind.
5. Extract first the juice from the pineapple.
6. Place the mango and cucumber into the juicer to extract their juices.
7. Juice the lemon last.
8. Transfer the extracts into your preferred container.
9. Stir or shake well before drinking.

- Expected Yield: 2 cups of juice
- Additional Health Benefits
- ❖ Improves the strength of the connective tissues of your skin
- ❖ Reduces the likelihood of swelling in your eyes

- ❖ Lowers water retention in your body
- ▪ Nutritional Value
  - ☐ Calories: 163
  - ☐ Carbohydrates: 52 grams
  - ☐ Sugars: 33 grams
  - ☐ Fiber: 6.9 grams
  - ☐ Protein: 3.9 grams
  - ☐ Fat: 0.53 grams
  - ☐ Sodium: 0.009 grams

- ○ *Cucumber Delight Juice*
  - ▪ Ingredients
    - ✓ 1 medium-sized cucumber
    - ✓ 1 celery stalk
    - ✓ 1 sprig fresh baby dill
  - ▪ Procedure
    1. Peel the cucumber, but keep its seeds intact.
    2. Chop the celery without removing its leaves.

3. Place both ingredients into the juicer.

4. Extract the juice.

5. Pour into a glass.

6. Stir well before garnishing it with dill on top.

- Expected Yield: 1.25 cups of juice

- Additional Health Benefits

❖ Keeps your whole body well hydrated

❖ Curbs your appetite, thus enabling you to lose extra weight

- Nutritional Value

☐ Calories: 31

☐ Carbohydrates: 8 grams

☐ Sugars: 4 grams

☐ Fiber: 2 grams

☐ Protein: 1.5 grams

☐ Fat: 0.12 grams

☐ Sodium: 0.05 grams

o *Papaya Surprise Juice*

- Ingredients
- ✓ ½ papaya
- ✓ 1 small pineapple
- ✓ 7 large strawberries
- Procedure

1. Remove the skin and seeds from the papaya.
2. Peel off the skin of the pineapple.
3. Chop the papaya and pineapple into cubes.
4. Place the papaya cubes, pineapple cubes, and strawberries into the juicer.
5. Extract the juice.
6. Pour into your favorite container.
7. Stir or shake well before drinking the juice.

- Expected Yield: 1.5 cups of juice
- Additional Health Benefits
  - ❖ Excellent in making the skin glow
  - ❖ Improves the health of your nails
- Nutritional Value

- Calories: 166
- Carbohydrates: 36 grams
- Sugars: 24 grams
- Fiber: 6.9 grams
- Protein: 4.3 grams
- Fat: 0.91 grams
- Sodium: 0.006 grams

Juices for Removing Environmental Toxins from the Body

Here are the five juice recipes that are excellent in flushing out the toxins from various organs of your body. If you are embarking on a juice fast, feel free to add any or all of these juices into your fasting plan.

- *Zesty Watermelon Juice*
- Ingredients
- 1 slice watermelon
- 1 slice cantaloupe
- 1 orange

- Procedure

1. Remove the peel and rinds from the watermelon and cantaloupe.
2. Remove the peel and pith of the orange.
3. Extract the juice from each ingredient, starting from the watermelon, and ending with the orange.
4. Transfer the juice into your preferred container.
5. Stir or shake well before drinking.

- Expected Yield: 1.5 cups of juice
- Additional Health Benefits

❖ Improves the quality of your vision

❖ Protects you from the common cold and flu

- Nutritional Value

❖ Calories: 164

❖ Carbohydrates: 45 grams

❖ Sugars: 36 grams

❖ Protein: 4.5 grams

❖ Fiber: 4.4 grams

- Fat: 0.83 grams
- Sodium: 0.027 gram

  - *Herbal Mango Juice*
    - Ingredients
      - 1 herbal tea bag of any kind
      - ½ mango
    - Procedure
      1. Remove the peel and pit from the mango.
      2. Extract the juice from the fruit.
      3. Brew the tea using hot water.
      4. Pour into your favorite teacup.
      5. Add ¼ cup of mango extract into 1 cup of tea.
      6. Stir well until the juice is well mixed with the tea.
    - Expected Yield: 2 cups of juice
    - Additional Health Benefits
      - Soothes the stomach
      - Makes you feel more energized

- Nutritional Value
  - Calories: 70
  - Carbohydrates: 18 grams
  - Sugars: 15 grams
  - Fiber: 2.1 grams
  - Protein: 1 gram
  - Fat: 0.23 gram
  - Sodium: 0.0045 gram

- *Refreshing Green Juice*
  - Ingredients

✓ 2 apples

✓ 1 cucumber

✓ 1 bunch parsley

✓ 1 bunch spinach

✓ ½ bunch celery

✓ ½ lemon

✓ ½ lime

- ✓ ½ ginger root
- Procedure

1. Remove the core and seeds of the apple, but keep its peel on.
2. Peel the cucumber, but keep its seeds.
3. Chop the celery along with its leaves.
4. Remove the peel off of the lemon and lime.
5. Extract the juice from spinach, cucumber, celery, parsley, ginger root, apples, lime, and lemon—one at a time, in this order.
6. Pour the extracts into your preferred container.
7. Stir or shake well to combine the juices.
8. Drink immediately.

- Expected Yield: 4 cups of juice
- Additional Health Benefits
- ✓ Quickens digestion
- ✓ Improves the flow and distribution of oxygen in the body
- Nutritional Value
- ☐ Calories: 225

- Carbohydrates: 38 grams
- Sugars: 28 grams
- Fiber: 17 grams
- Protein: 14 grams
- Fat: 2.6 grams
- Sodium: 0.461 gram

- *Beet-Orange Juice*
  - Ingredients
    - 1 beet
    - 2 oranges
  - Procedure
    1. Remove the greens from the beet.
    2. Peel off the skin and pith of the oranges.
    3. Juice the oranges first, then the beet.
    4. Transfer the extract into your favorite container.
    5. Stir and shake well before drinking the juice.
  - Expected Yield: 0.75 cup of juice

- Additional Health Benefits
- Increases your stamina by improving the blood flow into your muscles
- Boosts your immune system
- Nutritional Value
- Calories: 165
- Carbohydrates: 42 grams
- Sugars: 31 grams
- Fiber: 8.1 grams
- Protein: 4.5 grams
- Fat: 0.81 gram
- Sodium: 0.065 gram

- *Apple-Broccoli Juice*
- Ingredients
- 2 green apples
- 1 medium-sized orange
- ½ broccoli head

- ½ cup Italian parsley

- Procedure

1. Remove the core and seeds of the apples, but keeps their peel intact.
2. Peel off the skin and pit of the orange.
3. Chop the broccoli into florets.
4. Extract the juice from the apples and orange first.
5. Wrap the parsley on the broccoli florets before juicing them.
6. Transfer into your preferred container.
7. Stir or shake well before drinking.

- Expected Yield: 1.5 cups of juice
- Additional Health Benefits
  - Curbs your appetite
  - Protects the eyes from being damaged
    - Nutritional Value
      - Calories: 161
      - Carbohydrates: 47 grams

- Sugars: 32 grams
- Fiber: 8 grams
- Protein: 4.1 grams
- Fat: 0.89 gram
- Sodium: 0.031 gram

Juices for a Long and Healthy Life

The anti-aging properties of fresh juices from organic produce have long been recognized by several wellness experts. This is not entirely surprise because you may pack into a single juice all the vitamins, minerals, and antioxidants that are essential for longevity

Turn your juicer into the fountain of youth by following these recipes:

- *Mixed Berries Juice*
- Ingredients
- 1 bowl blackberries
- 1 bowl raspberries
- ½ lemon

- [x] ¼-inch ginger root

- Procedure

1. Remove the skin and pith of the lemon half.
2. Extract the juice from the blackberries and raspberries.
3. Juice the ginger root along with the lemon.
4. Pour into a glass or drinking bottle.
5. Stir or shake well to combine the juices.
6. Drink immediately.

- Expected Yield: 0.75 cups of juice

- Additional Health Benefits

- ❖ Lowers the risk of diabetes
- ❖ Protects the cells from free radicals

- Nutritional Value

- ☐ Calories: 268
- ☐ Carbohydrates: 63 grams
- ☐ Fiber: 32 grams
- ☐ Sugars: 27 grams
- ☐ Protein: 6.3 grams

- Fat: 3.1 grams
- Sodium: 0.007 gram

- *Heart-Friendly Juice*
  - Ingredients
    - 2 kale leaves
    - 1 celery stalk
    - 1 bunch spinach leaves
    - 1 cup wheatgrass
    - ½ lemon
  - Procedure
    1. Chop the celery stalk while keeping its leaves intact.
    2. Peel off the skin and pith from the lemon.
    3. Extract the juice the ingredients one by one in this order: celery, wheatgrass, spinach, kale, and lemon.
    4. Combine the juices in a glass or bottle.
    5. Stir or shake well.
    6. Consume immediately.

- Expected Yield: 1.25 cups of juice
- Additional Health Benefits
  - Increases the count of red blood cells
  - Reduces the risk of stroke by around 25%
- Nutritional Value
  - Calories: 72
  - Carbohydrates: 8 grams
  - Fiber: 4 grams
  - Protein: 3 grams
  - Sugars: 2 gram
  - Fat: 1 gram
  - Sodium: 0.1 gram

- *Anti-Inflammatory Juice*
  - Ingredients
    - 1 red apple
    - 1 cup red grapes
    - ½ lemon

- Procedure

1. Remove the core and seeds of the apple.
2. Remove the peel and pith of the lemon.
3. Extract the juice from the grapes, followed by the apple.
4. Juice the lemon last.
5. Pour into your favorite glass or bottle.
6. Stir well before drinking.

- Expected Yield: 1.25 cups of juice
- Additional Health Benefits

❖ Prevents joint pains
❖ Excellent at fighting off viral and bacterial infections

- Nutritional Value

☐ Calories: 102
☐ Carbohydrates: 48 grams
☐ Sugars: 39 grams
☐ Fiber: 3 grams
☐ Protein: 1.2 gram
☐ Fat: 0.54 gram

- *Fortifying Green Juice*
  - Ingredients
    - 2 romaine lettuce leaves
    - ½ broccoli head
    - 1 carrot
    - 1 bunch spinach
    - 1 garlic clove
    - ¼-inch ginger
  - Procedure
    1. Chop the broccoli into florets.
    2. In this order, extract the juice from the lettuce, spinach, broccoli, carrot, garlic, and ginger root.
    3. Transfer into your preferred container.
    4. Stir well to combine the extracts.
  - Expected Yield: 1.25 cups of juice
  - Additional Health Benefits
    - Relieves back pain

- ❖ Reduces the risk of bone degradation
- Nutritional Value
  - Calories: 186
  - Carbohydrates: 37 grams
  - Protein: 16 grams
  - Fiber: 14 grams
  - Sugars: 2.6 grams
  - Fat: 2.1 grams
  - Sodium: 0.352 gram

- *Carrot-Cantaloupe Surprise Juice*
- Ingredients
  - 2 carrots
  - 2 slices cantaloupe
  - 1 beet
- Procedure
  1. Peel off the skin of the carrots.
  2. Remove the rinds from the cantaloupe.

3. Chop off the greens of the beet.
4. Place the ingredients in your juicer.
5. Extract the juice.
6. Transfer into your preferred container.
7. Mix well the juices by stirring or shaking the juice.

- Expected Yield: 1.5 cups of juice
- Additional Health Benefits
  - Regulates blood pressure
  - Protects the eyes from damage due to excessive light exposure
- Nutritional Value
  - Calories: 251
  - Carbohydrates: 48 grams
  - Sugars: 33 grams
  - Fiber: 12 grams
  - Protein: 7.2 grams
  - Fat: 0.98 gram
  - Sodium: 0.20 gram

Green Smoothies

Are green juices the same thing as green smoothies?

Many beginners assume that they are one and the same. However, as you have learned in the earlier chapters of this book, juices and smoothies differ from one another in various ways—in terms of ingredients that you can use, preparation method, texture, and fiber content.

Keep in mind that standard juicers are not designed to handle smoothies. The produce that you would be using would only end up jamming the equipment. Instead, use a blender or a high-powered food processor instead.

Now, without further ado, here are the top five green smoothies that you give a try:

- *Blueberry Banana Green Smoothie*

  - Ingredients

    - 1 cup blueberries
    - 1 banana
    - ½ cup fresh spinach
    - ¼ cup fresh basil

- ✓ 2 cups non-dairy milk substitute
- Procedure

1. Chop the banana into 1-inch chunks.
2. Freeze the banana chunks for at least 24 hours.
3. Place all the ingredients, including the frozen banana chunks, into the blender.
4. Blend the ingredients until a smooth texture has been achieved.
5. Pour the smoothie into your preferred container.

- Expected Yield: 1 cup of smoothie
- Additional Health Benefits
  - ❖ Curbs your appetite by making you feel full for a long time
  - ❖ Improves and quickens digestion
  - ❖ Nutritional Value
    - Calories: 249
    - Carbohydrates: 50 grams
    - Sugars: 28 grams
    - Fat: 6 grams

- Protein: 5 grams

- *Minty Chocolate Green Smoothie*
  - Ingredients
    - 2 cups spinach leaves
    - ½ avocado
    - ¼ cup fresh mint leaves
    - 1 scoop chocolate protein powder
    - 1 tablespoon cacao nibs
    - 1 cup non-dairy milk substitute
    - 1 cup plain filtered water
    - A dash of stevia
    - Crushed ice (optional)
  - Procedure
    1. Place the spinach leaves, avocado, mint leaves, chocolate protein powder, cacao nibs, milk substitute, water, and stevia into the blender.
    2. Add crushed ice, if you prefer a cold smoothie.

3. Blend together the ingredients until the mixture has become thick and smooth.

4. Transfer into your preferred container.

- Expected Yield: 1 cup of smoothie
- Additional Health Benefits
  - Provides an energy boost
  - Suppresses your cravings for sweets and sugary drinks
- Nutritional Value
  - Calories: 365
  - Protein: 30 grams
  - Carbohydrates: 22 grams
  - Fat: 22 grams
  - Fiber: 10 grams
  - Sugars: 8 grams

- *Beet-Chard Green Smoothie*
  - Ingredients
    - 1 cup beets

- ✓ 1 bunch red chard
- ✓ 1 cup crushed ice
- ✓ ½ cup fresh apple juice
- ✓ ½ cup almond milk
- ✓ 1 teaspoon natural sweetener of your choice
- ✓ 1 teaspoon pure vanilla extract

- Procedure

1. Peel and chop the beets into cubes
2. Steam lightly the beet cubes.
3. Chop the red chard into smaller bits. Include the stems for your smoothie.
4. Place all the ingredients into the blender.
5. Mix the ingredients until the texture has become rich and creamy.
6. Transfer the smoothie into your favorite container.

- Expected Yield: 1 cup of smoothie
- Additional Health Benefits
- ❖ Improves your physical performance

- ❖ Boosts your immune system
- Nutritional Value
  - Calories: 270
  - Carbohydrates: 39 grams
  - Protein: 20 grams
  - Fiber: 5 grams
  - Fat: 4 grams

  Juicing Tip: For the sweetener required by this recipe, opt for raw honey, maple syrup, agave nectar, or stevia. These natural sweeteners would prevent a spike up of your blood sugar.

- *Zesty Green Smoothie*
- Ingredients
  - ✓ 1 cup fresh baby spinach
  - ✓ 1 kiwi
  - ✓ 1 small-sized cucumber
  - ✓ ½ green apple
  - ✓ ½ cup lemon-flavored seltzer or sparkling water

- ✓ 1 tablespoon lemon juice
- ✓ plain water (as needed)
- Procedure

1. Scoop out the flesh of the kiwi from its peel.
2. Remove the seeds from the apple.
3. Place the baby spinach, kiwi, cucumber, green apple, and lemon juice into the blender.
4. Blend the ingredients together until everything has been evenly mixed.
5. Add water, as needed, to achieve the desired texture.
6. Transfer the contents of the blender into your preferred container.
7. Pour the sparkling water or seltzer on top of the blended ingredients.
8. Stir well to combine.
9. Consume immediately.

- Expected Yield: 1 cup of smoothie
- Additional Health Benefits
- ❖ Hydrates the whole body

- ❖ Suppresses infections and inflammations
- Nutritional Value
  - Calories: 95
  - Carbohydrates: 23 grams
  - Fiber: 5 grams
  - Protein: 2 grams

- *Pineapple Kale Green Smoothie*
  - Ingredients
    - ✓ 1 small pineapple
    - ✓ 1 bunch kale
    - ✓ 3 sprigs cilantro
    - ✓ ¾ cup non-fat Greek yoghurt
    - ✓ 1 teaspoon agave nectar
    - ✓ 1 teaspoon fresh lime juice
    - ✓ 1 teaspoon chia seeds
    - ✓ A dash of chili powder
  - Procedure

1. Peel off the skin of the pineapple.
2. Cut the pineapple into chunks.
3. Place pineapple chunks, kale, cilantro, yoghurt, agave nectar, lime juice, and chia seeds into the blender.
4. Blend the ingredients together until the texture has become smooth.
5. Pour the smoothie your preferred container.
6. Sprinkle chili powder on top of the smoothie.

- Expected Yield: 1 cup of smoothie
- Additional Health Benefits
  - Makes you feel full for an extended period of time
  - Speeds up your digestion
- Nutritional Value
  - Calories: 192
  - Carbohydrates: 26 grams
  - Protein: 19 grams
  - Sugar: 19 grams
  - Fiber: 3.4 grams

- Fat: 2 grams

For those with more experience in juicing, feel free to experiment with the recipes below by substituting the ingredients with your preferred produce or adding juice boosters into the mix.

However, for beginners, it is best to practice first by recreating the recipes given in this chapter. Doing so would enable you to get a better feel of the juicing process itself, and your personal preferences when it comes to taste and texture.

Chapter 8 – Enhancing Your Juice Cleansing Experience

Unlocking the benefits of juicing can be a lot easier when you are actually enjoying what you are doing. You do not have to force yourself to drink juices and smoothies that gross you out. Numerous herbs and spices can improve upon the taste and nutritional content of your beverage.

You also do not have just wait things out until you feel the effects of juicing on your body. Exercising while in a juice fast hastens the process of losing weight, fighting off diseases, and achieving good health.

In this chapter, you will learn the various ways to enhance your juicing experience. Discover the best herbs and spices that you can use to upgrade your juices and smoothies. Find out also the kinds of exercises that you can without having to spend long, grueling hours at the gym.

Applying these strategies to your juice cleanse would not only make it a more enjoyable activity, but also a more rewarding journey towards a long and healthy life.

Enhancing the Flavor and Nutritional Value of Your Juices

Much like in cooking, you can take things up a notch by adding your favorite herbs and spices into your juice. Aside from adding a new layer of flavor, these juice enhancers are packed with their own sets of nutrients as well.

Here is a list of the top herbs and spices, and how each will elevate your juice experience.

1. Basil

- Boosts the immune system
- Fights off bacterial infections
- Excellent source of Vitamin A, Vitamin K, and calcium

2. Cilantro

- Reduces the amount of bad cholesterol, while increasing the good cholesterol in your blood
- Controls the level of blood sugar
- Prevents bacterial infections, particularly those caused by salmonella

3. Cinnamon

- Improves the condition of the heart and colon
- Boosts the defense mechanisms of the immune system
- Promotes efficient blood clotting
- Fights off fungi and bacteria

- Enhances brain performance

4. Ginger

- Relieves issues related to the stomach and intestines, such as excessing gas, motion sickness, and morning sickness
- Lowers the risk of getting the common cold
- Reduces the pain and swelling caused by arthritis
- Prevents the growth and development of ovarian cancer

5. Horseradish

- Eliminates acne
- Relieves headache, sinusitis joint pain, muscle aches, and urinary tract infection
- Protects you from the cold virus and the flu virus
- Lowers the risk of various respiratory problems, especially those that are caused by bacterial infections

6. Lemongrass

- Boosts your energy levels
- Promotes a faster healing process
- Aids in removing toxins from your body
- Regulates your blood sugar levels

- Increases the amount of oxygen in the blood

7. Oregano

- Reduces the risk of cancer
- Protects your body from bacterial infections

8. Peppermint

- Promotes quick digestions
- Soothes pain in the stomach and intestines
- Reduces the intensity of respiratory symptoms caused by an allergic reaction or asthma
- Kills different types of bacteria, such as salmonella, Staphylococcus aureus, and E. coli

Enhancing the Benefits of Juice Cleansing

Not many people know that juicing and cardio exercises go well with one another. Many experts actually consider this combination as the quickest way to lose weight.

In case you are not familiar with the concept, cardio exercises refer to a set of low-intensity physical aerobic activities. Common examples include walking, jogging, and hiking.

These cardio exercises help you lose weight during a fast by speeding up the oxidation process—or the burning off of your excess fat stores. Fasting itself triggers this, but coupling it with a light workout could increase significantly the amount of fat that you can eliminate.

Aside from promoting lipolysis, or the process of releasing fatty acids to convert them into energy, cardio exercise while in a juice cleanse can help you achieve the following health benefits:

- Reduced stress levels
- Fewer inflammations in the body
- Stronger and denser bones
- Reduced risk of diabetes
- Better cardiovascular healthier
- Lower blood pressure
- More stable mood
- Higher libido

Experts suggest that the best time for cardio exercises is upon waking up in the morning. While in a fast, you can start off by drinking a cup of herbal tea or a juice made from tea leaves extract. This would give you enough nutrition to get by the cardio exercise without damaging your body.

In terms of the kind of cardio exercise that you should be doing, keep things simple by opting for whatever would work for your current responsibilities and schedule.

You do not have to get a subscription at the gym. You do not also have to buy special exercise equipment for this. Just by going outside for a 20 to 30-minute brisk walk would be enough to unlock the additional benefits of cardio to your juice fast.

If you end up choosing brisk walking as your main cardio, make sure to use minimalistic footwear. Unlike in running, where you are encouraged to wear running shoes, the intensity of walking is not enough to fully exercise the muscles in your feet and lower legs.

Should you find walking to be a bit too boring for you, feel free to try out other ways to get your blood pumping. Casual sports can be considered as a form of low-intensity cardio exercise. For example, playing frisbee at the park would still be beneficial for your body. If you enjoy golfing more, then go out and play a few rounds with your friends.

The important thing is that the activity would not be too intense for your body. Remember, you are essentially in a fasted state. Your body would not appreciate tiresome and strenuous activities, given the lack of solid foods in your current diet. Keep things light and fun, and soon you would be able to feel the difference that fasted cardio can bring to your health.

Enhancing Your Coping Mechanisms for the Side-Effects of Juice Cleansing

1. Drink more water.

Just because you are drinking juices and smoothies does not mean that you would have to forego drinking water altogether. Experts recommend drinking the recommended amount of water per day even while you are in the middle of a juice fast.

You have to be careful about ensuring the balance of fluids in your body though. Keeping this at an optimal level would help you:

- eliminate wastes from various organs of the body, such as the skin, lungs, kidneys, and colon-related;
- regulate the production and release of hormones;
- transport nutrients across different parts of the body in an efficient manner.

Too little water would lead to dehydration. When your body lacks water, even if you are drinking juices and smoothies regularly, you would suffer from the following symptoms:

- Headaches or migraines
- Depression
- Pain in the intestines
- Joint pain and swelling
- Chronic hunger
- High blood pressure

If you have not yet noticed, many of these symptoms bear similarities with those that you might experience when your body is undergoing withdrawal from solid foods, sugars, and/or caffeine.

As such, expect the severity and frequency of these symptoms to increase if you become dehydrated while you are preparing or already engaging in a juice fast.

You might already be familiar with the effects of dehydration on your body. However, you should also be aware of the probable negative effects of too much water on your health.

According to medical experts, drinking too much water on a short period of time would lead to water intoxication. Symptoms of over-hydration includes nausea, headache, and dizziness. This can escalate to seizures and coma, if the sodium in your blood becomes too diluted.

How would you be able to tell if you are drinking too little or too much of water? The simplest way, with no cost involved at all, is by monitoring frequency and color of your urine.

Studies show an average person who is well-hydrated urinates about six to eight times per day. Therefore, if you urinate more than the eight times each day, you should hold back yourself from drinking too much water. However, urinating less than six times a day should be regarded as warning that you are not drinking enough water.

The color of the urine should be light yellow. Any darker shade than that may be considered as a sign as a sign of dehydration. On the other hand, almost clear urines might be an indicator that you are getting too much water in your system.

Aside from the amount of water you should be drinking, you must also be mindful of its quality. One of the main reasons you are going through a juice fast is to eliminate the traces of environmental toxins in your body. Therefore, the last thing you would want to do is unwittingly ingest more toxins whenever you drink water.

For many people, tap water is the most accessible and cheapest source of water. However, there is a probability that it is not actually safe for drinking. Studies show that tap water can easily be contaminated with chemical pollutants, heavy metals, radiological substances, and water parasites.

As such, you should avoid drinking tap water unless you are absolutely sure of its quality. Look for other viable sources for you to ensure that you are drinking safe and pure water.

One of the popular options available nowadays is the installation of a water filtration system at home. It is best to get your tap water tested first though so that you would be able to identify what kinds of particles and chemicals must be filtered out from your water.

Do not replace tap with bottled water though. The packaging itself contains pollutants that can not only adversely affect the environment, but your own body as well.

Many manufacturers use BPA (Bisphenol A) and phthalates in their plastic bottles. Even at little amounts, these chemicals can be harmful to your health. Aside from causing various types of diseases, the chemicals can disrupt the hormonal balance inside your body.

To keep you from having these additional problems, opt for sustainable water filtration system in your home instead. If your budget permits, it would be best if you could extend this system beyond just your drinking water, but also to your cooking water and bathing water.

2. Eliminate the sources of toxins around you.

As explained earlier, you should minimize the amount of toxins that your body is exposed to, not just while you are on a juice fast, but every single day. Doing so would reduce the pains, swelling, and diseases that you might suffer from.

Furthermore, this would also enhance the effects of juicing cleansing on your body and mind. Studies show that removing these sources out of your home would boost your immune system, make you look younger and slimmer, and enable you to perform better at both physical and mental activities.

To eliminate the potential sources of toxins around you, you must first take note of your surroundings. Identify things inside your home that may contain pollutants that are harmful for your body.

Here is a list of common sources of toxins to get you started, and what you may do to remove or minimize them.

- Cleaning Agents

Common household cleaning chemicals, such as bleach, air fresheners, and drain cleaners, contain lots of toxins in them. These can enter your body when you inhale their fumes while using them. You should avoid this at all cost because these toxins cause significant damage to the nervous system.

Fortunately, the market is not full of cleaning agents that contain little to no toxins at all. You may also try making your own cleaning chemicals by using ingredients that you can easily find in the supermarket. For example, vinegar and lemon have been used for centuries as all-natural stain removers.

- Padded furniture, carpets, and rugs

You are exposed to your household furniture day and night, thereby making them significant contributors to the amount of toxins that enter your body.

For instance, the foam in padded furniture and mattresses emits lots of toxic fumes especially when they are newly bought. Air them out first for a day or two before attempting to use them.

Furthermore, some carpets and rugs are also sprayed heavily with insecticides to prevent an infestation of tiny insects and dust mites. To keep these toxins at a minimum, opt for carpets that are made of natural fibers such as jute and sisal. Foregoing a latex backing would also lessen the fumes coming out from the carpet or rug.

- Indoor Air

Most people stay indoors for more than half of the day. Therefore, the quality of air inside the house can significantly affect one's health.

Studies show that in many households, the air is filled with almost twice as much pollutants than those found outside. Such an observation is likely due to the various sources of toxins present in a much smaller space.

To lessen the amount of toxins in the air you breathe at home, you should open your windows for at least a couple of hours per day. This would allow the fresh air from the outside to come in, thus ensuring smooth air flow inside the house.

If it is too cold to open the windows, then you may use an air purifier instead. This would filter out the dust, toxic fumes, smoke, bacteria, molds, and pollens that are present in the air. You can find one that would fit in your budget at the local malls and appliance stores.

Aside from your home, toxins may also come from the various things that you apply onto yourself. The skin, after all, is an organ that is porous enough to allow these chemicals and pollutants to get into your bloodstream.

Protect your skin from these toxins by following these tips on the quality of body care products that you should get instead.

- Toothpaste

Some popular brands of toxins contain artificial sweeteners, and chemicals that can be harmful to your health. Rather these commercially produced variants, opt for the natural brands that can be bought in health and wellness stores.

- Shampoo

Spend time in reading the label at the back of a shampoo bottle. If you cannot recognize most of its ingredients, then that variant most likely contains various chemicals—some of which may be detrimental to your body.

Again, look for shampoos made of natural ingredients instead. More and more organic brands are also entering the supermarkets and malls, so be sure to check those out.

- Deodorizers and antiperspirants

Avoid deodorizers and antiperspirants that contain aluminum. Studies have linked this substance to breast cancer. After all, the armpits are close to your breasts. Even if you are careful at applying deodorizers and antiperspirants on yourself, there would still be the risk of exposing your breast tissues to this chemical.

Given this, organic and natural variants of deodorizers and antiperspirants are the ideal choices for both men and women.

- Makeup and moisturizing creams

These skin care products are notoriously known for containing lots of potentially harmful chemicals. The best way to avoid such toxins is to buy the unscented variants with no petrochemicals in them. Many makeup companies make this as their selling point, so you would not have a hard looking for toxin-free makeup and moisturizing creams that suitable for your skin.

Though these guidelines may seem incredibly limiting, rest assured that the recent trend for healthier and eco-friendlier products continually grows day by day. As such, the toxin-free options that you may choose from would also widen over time.

At this point, just be sure to read and research every product that you would use at home and on yourself. Doing so would prevent you from having to frequently go through the ill side-effects of detoxification on your body.

3. Minimize the stress in your life.

    The body is under significant strain while you are in a juice fast. Fortunately, the human body has evolved to effectively handle light to moderate stress. The internal processes adapt to the situation you are in by changing the way glucose is released in your bloodstream, burning more fat for energy, and making you more sensitive to insulin.

    Since your body is already experiencing some form of stress, you should try to eliminate or keep away the external stressors in your life. The less stress imposed upon you, the more resources could be allocated for more beneficial activities, such as burning off more fats, healing your body, and regenerating replacements for the damaged cells.

    Ignoring this advice by letting yourself become stressed out for a long period of time can lead to various health conditions, such as:

    - Anxiety
    - Depression
    - Elevated heart rate

- Fatigue
- High blood pressure
- Hormonal imbalance
- Infertility
- Memory problems
- Obesity

To keep yourself from having to suffer these conditions, and to lead a happy and healthy life, you should stay away from the potential sources of stress. Try to remove yourself from situations that only will cause you stress.

That is, of course, easier said than done for most people. However, you have to make an active choice to seek a relatively stress environment. Do not hesitate to ask for the help and support of your family, friends, and co-workers in realizing this goal.

4. Get enough rest and sleep.

Whether or not you are on a fast, the right amount of good-quality sleep is essential for achieving good health. Sleep does matter more while fasting because it allows the body to recover and regenerate faster. Furthermore, you are less likely to feel hunger while you are asleep, thus making fasting a lot easier to handle.

Nowadays, however, there are plenty of factors that can keep you from getting enough sleep. The simple use of your cellphone while in bed can rob you of your recovery time. As such, many people suffer from the effects of sleep deprivation.

Depriving yourself of sleep while in a juice fast can be disastrous for your health and wellbeing. Studies show that this may lead to the following outcomes:

- Weight Gain

    Without enough sleep, the hormones in your body would begin to shift, thus altering your appetite as well. In time, you will notice yourself craving for more sugar in your diet.

    The problem is compounded by the fact that sleep deprivation also affects how well your body would metabolize sugar. Being in this state for too long would lead to slow metabolism, thus making you gain more weight than usual.

    On the other hand, research shows that you may lose up to 14 pounds per year just by increasing the duration of sleep by 1 hour per night.

- Compromised Immune System

    The natural defense mechanisms of your body lowers down whenever you miss out on your sleep. As a result, you would become more vulnerable to different types of illnesses, ranging from minor ones, such as the common cold, to chronic health conditions, such as cancer and neurodegenerative diseases.

- Weakened Regenerative Capabilities

Aside from the immune system, your ability to regenerate cells and heal damaged tissues would become less effective as well. This particularly affect your brain tissues and neurons, thus negatively affecting your memory, creativity, and ability to concentrate on your tasks.

- Various Types of Heart Diseases

When your body can no longer process sugar the right way, you would develop insulin resistance. This condition can then lead to the conversion of the carbohydrates in your body into bad cholesterol. Increased water retention can also cause high blood pressure, thus putting you at a higher risk for developing cardiovascular diseases.

- Premature Aging

Sleep deprivation reduces the production and release of growth hormones that are essential for repairing damaged tissues, rejuvenating cells, and ensuring optimal bone health. Without these hormones, you would notice early appearance of the various signs of aging across your body.

The effects of sleep deprivation do not simply go away by making up for the sleep you have lost the following day. They accumulate over time because the body is not adapted to being in this state frequently. As such, you would just feel even more tired, and more prone to various illnesses and obesity.

The best way to prevent this from happening to you is by making a habit out of good sleeping practices, and training your body to follow a natural sleeping cycle.

Referred to as the circadian rhythm, this is the key to getting good-quality sleep without much effort from your part. Applying this concept into your lifestyle prior to engaging in a juice fast would help you lower the stressors in your life, and thus enhance the benefits that you may expect from the fast itself.

To help you adapt the natural sleeping cycle, here are some important tips on getting the enough good-quality sleep every day.

- Avoid drinking caffeinated drinks in the evening.

  Caffeine makes it harder for your body to get ready for sleep. It also reduces the duration of deep sleep that you would get.

If you really want to consume caffeine during this time of day, make sure that you do so at least 3 hours before your bedtime. This would enable your body to completely process the caffeine, thereby minimizing its effects on your sleep.

- Do not consume alcoholic drinks before going to bed.

    Though alcohol can help you fall asleep faster, it would significantly lower down the quality of sleep that you can get. It would prevent you from falling into a deep sleep and entering the REM (Rapid Eye Movement) phase of your sleep.

- Eliminate all sources of light from your bedroom.

    The human body produces melatonin—an essential hormone for sleeping while it is in the darkness. Therefore, when there is any source of light in your bedroom, the production of this hormone would be reduced or stopped altogether. This would make it even harder for you to fall asleep.

    Turning off the lights in your bedroom is not enough when light from the outside can still enter your sleeping space. To effectively block them off, install blackout curtains or shades on the windows of your bedroom.

Make sure that fabric or material is thick enough that you cannot see the outline of any figure from the other side. There should also be no visible gaps in between the curtains or shades because light from the outside would continue to stream into the room.

- Make sure that your bedroom is well-ventilated.

  For most people, the ideal temperature for the bedroom is 68 ºF (20 ºC). However, if that is not comfortable for you, then feel free to alter the temperature to your liking. Just make sure that it is on the cooler side because the body is adapted to such an environment.

  Some people use electric fans and air coolers to maintain a good circulation of air in the room. There are also others who use air purifiers to ensure the quality of air they breathe in while asleep.

- Refrain from using your personal devices before going to bed.

  Avoid using your phone, tablets, or computer at least one before your bedtime. You should also avoid watching the television because it would keep you from falling asleep.

  The lights emitted by these devices hamper the production of melatonin in your body. You are also less likely to feel calm and relaxed when you browse social media posts, or watch the news while you are in bed.

Turn off these devices at night to prevent them from negatively affecting your sleep. In case you need to set an alarm for the following morning, consider using a traditional alarm clock rather than your cellphone or tablet.

- Go to sleep at the same time every night.

Doing so would train your body to naturally go to sleep at a certain time. According to experts, the best schedule for most people is to sleep by 10 at night, and wake up by 7 in the morning.

During this period of time, the body is at its peak of repairing itself. More growth hormones are also produced during the early parts of the morning

Waking up at in time for the sunrise would also help you regulate the production of other hormones that are important for your body. This would keep your health at an optimal condition for the rest of the day.

Sleeping is as important as detoxifying the body. No matter how well you eat and how much you exercise, your health would not significantly improve without getting enough rest and sleep.

Chapter 9 – Ending Your Juice Cleanse the Right Way

If you think that you can just simply jump in and out of a juice cleanse, then you would be putting your health at risk. Though planning for a juice fast tends to be much longer and more detailed, transitioning your body from being in a fasted state is a delicate process as well.

It requires some advance planning as well because there are a lot of things to consider and observe during the transition period. At this point, your body would be at its most sensitive, so exercising great care in the food you would be eating, and activities that you would do.

The challenge of breaking a juice fast stems from the need to maintain homeostasis, or balance in your body. During a fast, you are essentially in survival mode. Your intake of calories would be limited; hence the body would do its best to strategically use whatever resources you have on hand.

The result can be observed in the expected benefits from a juice fast. For example, you would lose more weight, and be cleansed of the toxins inside your body.

Being in survival mode would also influence multiple systems in your body, including but are not limited to your defense mechanisms, hormone production, metabolism, and digestion.

In other words, your body would function differently than when you are eating solid foods. Transitioning from this state back to your normal ways becomes harder the longer you fast because your body would grow accustomed to its altered conditions and functions.

Rushing yourself back to your regular eating patterns would cause health complications, such as:

- Nausea

- Heartburn

- Bloating

- Diarrhea

- Constipation

Some people who failed to shift themselves gradually also experience physical and mental fatigue.

Therefore, to prevent suffering from these symptoms, and to gain a holistic understanding of this health improvement strategy, you must learn the proper way of breaking a juice fast.

Here are the most important tips that you have to keep in mind when preparing ahead for your post-cleanse diet and activities.

- On the first day after you have completed your juice fast, eat only fresh fruits, vegetables, and nuts.

  If you do not enjoy eating vegetables raw, then you may blanch or lightly steam them instead. Some recommend roasting vegetables as well, but be careful not to overcook them.

  Pureeing or incorporating vegetables into soup is another great way of reintroducing solids into your diet. Opt for clear or thin soup bases instead of rich and creamy ones to avoid straining your stomach.

  Experts suggest eating at least 5 small servings of raw or steamed vegetables per day. Space your feeding times throughout the day so as to keep the strain on your stomach to a minimum.

  For fruits, limit yourself to only 2 small servings each day. This would help in easing your body out of its fasted state. The insoluble fibers in the fruits you eat would also hasten your digestion and bowel movements.

- Keep your portion sizes small so as to prevent shocking your digestive system.

Your digestive system has been "resting" for majority of the time spent on a juice fast. As such, you should go easy when it comes to eating again solid foods.

- Limit your intake of coffee or any caffeinated beverage.

  Giving up on coffee before and during your juice cleanse is a necessary step of the process. Continuing to do so right after a juice fast is not be a strict requirement, but it is highly recommended by many juicing experts.

  The high acidic content of caffeinated drinks can be tough to handle for a stomach that has been resting for the past few days. However, if you are keen on putting them back on your regular diet, then do so in small, incremental step.

  Start by drinking around ¼ cup of coffee without sugar. Then, increase the amount by another ¼ the following day. If you feel any discomfort in your stomach, stop drinking and let your body rest for a bit longer.

- You may use this adjustment period to observe the reactions of your body to certain types of food.

  List down in a journal the foods and beverages that you are adding into your meals. Then, record your observations in the same journal to keep better track of your notes on how the food affected your energy level, and digestion.

- Take note also if you have developed any kind of symptom or allergic reaction from the food or drink you have consumed.

  The detox process may cause significant alterations to your body, so the best time to assess these changes is the adjustment period.

- Day by day, reintroduce other types of food and beverages into your diet, but do not revert back to eating processed foods, refined sugars, and dairy products.

  Your stomach should be ready for regular meals by the fifth day after finishing a multiple-day fast.

  Eat only lean proteins if you are going to eat meat. Avoid fatty cuts because this would be too much for your sensitive stomach to handle.

  Instead, opt for healthy fats from fruits, vegetables, and nuts. Good sources include avocados, almonds, and olive oil.

  When it comes to grains, always choose whole grains, even if have already successfully transitioned yourself from a juice fast to your regular diet. They provide more carbohydrates without raising too much your blood sugar levels.

- Avoid sugars as much as possible.

If you have to, use only natural sweeteners that are mostly plant-based—for example, honey, maple syrup, agave nectar, and stevia.

Refined sugars can hard for the liver to break down. Furthermore, this type of sweetener invites more cravings rather than satisfy your hunger. As such, try your best to stay away from food products and beverages that are high in refined sugars.

- Remember to drink plenty of water each day.

If plain water becomes too boring or tiresome for you, switch things up by enjoying a cup of hot tea. Water infused with fruits slices can also be great alternatives for keeping you hydrated during this period.

- Say no to alcohol.

If you enjoy drinking alcoholic beverages, continue your abstinence for at least 7 days more after you have ended your juice fast.

During this period, your liver is still undergoing active detoxification. Imbibing alcohol before the process has been completed would effectively put a stop to the removal of impurities from this body organ.

Maximize the benefits of a juice cleanse by giving your liver as much as it needs to rest and detoxify.

- Move your body.

    Start by doing simple exercises for your body, such as walking and stretching. Remember, your energy levels are not as high as when you were consuming more calories, so it is best to keep things light.

    Once you have begun eating more solid foods again, then you may proceed with more strenuous exercises, such as swimming or playing a casual game of basketball. This would help you sustain the momentum of the detoxification process within your body.

- Perform other activities that will make you sweat.

    The skin is considered as the largest detoxification organ in the human body. To support its cleansing process even after you have finished a juice detox, go to a sauna, hot bath, or steam room to keep yourself sweating without expending so much energy.

    By doing so, you would be able to remove more toxins from your body as you transition back to your regular activities.

- Meditate.

    This can be helpful in managing your stress levels. Letting yourself be carried away by the demands and difficulties of your life would only make this period more delicate than it should be.

Meditation helps you focus on the positive aspects of your life. It would also remind of your reasons for engaging in a juice fast in the first place.

- Rest, and get enough quality sleep.

Resting and sleeping are the best ways to relieve yourself of the stress and discomfort that you would be feeling during this period. This would also enable your body to prepare itself for the new set of changes that is coming your way.

If you have followed the advice regarding the natural circadian rhythm of the body, then try to sustain the sleeping habits and patterns that you have learned and practiced during your juice fast.

To further support you through the post-cleansing phase of your journey, here is a menu guide that you can follow while you are transitioning back to your regular diet:

Day 1

Eat only three small meals that may be composed by any combination of the following:

- Fresh vegetable salad, or steamed vegetables of any kind

- Vegetable soup or puree

- Carrot sticks, turnip sticks, or celery stalks

- Sliced fresh fruits of any kind

- Nuts or seeds

- Coconut oil or extra-virgin olive oil

- Mild herbs and spices, but only to slightly flavor your food

Make sure to drink plain water or a warm cup of herbal tea before, during, and after your meals.

You should also begin taking notes of the sensations caused by these foods to your body. Remember to do so as well for every succeeding day from this point on.

Day 2

Once more, limit yourself to only three small portions of the following foods throughout the day.

- Steamed or roasted vegetables of any kind

- Starchy root crops, such as potatoes and sweet potatoes

- Brown rice, Adlai rice, or quinoa

- Sliced fresh fruits of any kind

- Nuts or seeds

- Beans or legumes

- Plant-based oils

- Mild herbs and spices as flavorings for your food

Again, do not forget to consume plenty of fluids from morning until before you go to bed.

Day 3

You may begin reintroducing some forms of dairy into your diet. However, you still have to observe the 3-meal rule for this transition period. You may consider eating any of the following foods:

- Fresh vegetable salad, or steamed or roasted vegetables, or vegetable soup
- Brown rice, Adlai rice, quinoa
- Non-fat, unsweetened plain yoghurt
- Organic eggs
- Sliced fresh fruits
- Nuts or seeds
- Beans or legumes
- Vegetable oil, extra-virgin olive oil, or coconut oil
- Herbs and spices

If you cannot find organic eggs or if they are outside your budget, then do not make do with commercially produced eggs. They may be laden with antibiotics and other chemicals that can be harsh for your sensitive stomach.

You should also keep yourself well hydrated by drinking plain water, fruit-infused water, and herbal teas.

Day 4

At this point, your stomach is ready for lean meats, light poultry meat, and fish. Here are the suggested types of food that you may eat during this day.

- Fresh vegetable salads, soups, or puree
- Steamed or roasted vegetables
- Tofu
- Lean cuts of beef, pork, or lamb
- Tuna, salmon, or mackerel
- Chicken breast
- Brown rice, Adlai rice, or quinoa
- Nuts or seeds
- Edamame beans
- Organic, unsweetened plain yoghurt
- Organic eggs

- Plant-based oils

Since you have started eating more solid foods, keep in mind that you should take your time in chewing them well. Doing so would aid and speed up your digestive system

Water and tea would also boost your digestion. Remember to drink plenty throughout the day.

Day 5

Your stomach is now ready to digest a normal, well-balanced diet. This means that even though you are out of the transition period, you should still avoid consuming unhealthy foods and beverages, especially those that are high in refined sugars, salt, and trans-fat.

If you want to keep off the weight you have lost during the juice cleanse, then avoid drinking caffeine and alcoholic drinks for as long as you can. Your water weight can easily come back when you adapt such practices once more.

Make sure to go over your notes about the effects of the foods that you have eaten. Those pieces of information are valuable in sustaining the health improvements that juice cleansing have given to you for a longer period of time. When you have the time, you may share these observations with your physician so that he/she can better interpret these data for you.

Conclusion

I'd like to thank you and congratulate you for transiting my lines from start to finish.

I hope this book was able to help you to convince you to pursue juicing as a way of improving your health.

The next step is to apply the most valuable lessons and tips provided in this ultimate guide on juicing. As a final reminder, here are the important points that you must carry with you, and share with others:

- Losing weight, preventing chronic diseases, and reversing the signs of aging do not have to be complicated.

You do not have to rely on expensive gears, creams, or supplements that promise to do all sorts of things to your body.

Juicing can be as easy and simple as you want it to be. It can help you achieve such goals without requiring a lot of time, effort, and money from you. It can help you:

  - get rid of the dangerous toxins inside your body;
  - speed up and improve your digestion;
  - burn off your excess fat;
  - increase your energy levels;

- improve your mental capacity;
- brighten up your skin;
- promote the growth and development of your bones; and
- delay the process of aging.

  Though there are various risks associated with juicing, there are also several ways to minimize or eliminate completely these potential dangers to your health.

- There are tons of fruits and vegetables that could help you achieve your health goals.

  Having a lot of produce to choose from may paralyze others from pursuing juicing altogether. But with this comprehensive guide, you do not have to worry at all about making the wrong selections.

  Whether you want to shake off your excess belly fat, or if you want to feel more energized, there is surely a produce that could make you satisfy your needs. Everything you need to know about the best fruits and vegetables for juicing—including their nutritional content and potential health benefits—has been given to you on a detailed but easily digestible list.

- The right juicer for you depends on your personal needs, goals, and budget.

Do not be blinded by all the shiny features and high-tech accessories of a juice. The perfect juicer for you might not have to be the top-of-the-line model.

In this guide, you have learned about the features of the different types of juicer—all of which comes with their own advantages and disadvantages. Knowing is only one step though, so this book has taken a step further by showing you exactly how to properly assess the available juicers in the market.

Since there are literally thousands of juicers to choose from, I have also given you valuable tips on how to get the best deals, and which models are considered by many juicing enthusiasts as the best in their respective categories.

- Creating your juices at home can be easier by setting up a simple but functional juicing station.

Juicing is both an art and a science. Practice this in the comforts of your own kitchen by having the right tools and kitchen supplies at your disposable.

As you can tell by the list I have given you, you do not have to buy complicated machines and pricey accessories to set up a good juicing station. If you know your needs well, then you can just focus on getting the essentials for yourself.

Your juicing station is not complete without a nice set of juice boosters. Lining up your shelf with these recommended natural additives would help you kick up the nutritional value of your self-made juices.

- Detoxing the body through juices and smoothies can give your body a much needed break.

    Though the human body is naturally equipped with parts that actively filter out toxins, you should still support them by allowing them enough time to rest and recover.

    Some people may try to dissuade you from doing this, especially given the significant known health risks of going through a detox. However, if you have sought the approval of your doctor first, and you can really commit yourself to this activity, then juice cleansing would be a life-altering experience for you.

- Juice cleansing does not have to be boring, tiring, or painful.

    You can take a more proactive approach by following our tips on enhancing the flavor of your juice. Remember to use those herbs and spices lightly at first though since they can be quite tasty and overpowering.

    Enhancing the benefits of a juice cleanse can also be done to get the most out of your time and effort to detox your body. The great thing about this is that you do not have to force yourself to go to the gym or to workout at all. You can enjoy better benefits from your juice fast if you would limit yourself only to light activities.

With the right strategy and mindset, the pains and discomforts of going through a juice fast can be minimized, too. Becoming a healthier version of you should not be a hellish experience at all.

Juicing means caring for your personal health. Aiming for anything other than that could lead to disastrous consequences for your general wellbeing.

- Safely end your juice cleanse by being patient with yourself.

Many beginners fail to take the final step into consideration, especially when they were too excited to see the benefits of juicing on their body. Fortunately, this book is written to guide you through the entire process.

Keep in mind the things you should do, and the practices that you should avoid after going through a juice fast. Don't let your time and effort go to waste just because you cannot control of your urges for a little bit longer.

As a final note, I want you to try and make juicing an intimate experience for you. While you should take heed of the various tips and strategies explained in this guide, you should also set aside some time to listen to your personal needs and preferences as well.

By doing so, you would be able to better identify the juicing practices and recipes that are going to work best for you.

I know you could have picked any number of books to read, but you picked this book and for that I am extremely grateful.

I hope that it added at value and quality to your everyday life. If so, it would be really nice if you could share this book with your friends and family by posting to Facebook and Twitter.

If you enjoyed this book and found some benefit in reading this, I'd like to hear from you and hope that you could take some time to post a review. I want you, the reader, to know that your review is very important and so, if you'd like to leave a review, all you have to do is click here and away you go. I wish you all the best in your future success!

Thank you and good luck!

Madison Fuller

Resources Page

Crocker, P. (2016, March 26). A Brief History of Juicing - dummies. Retrieved October 28, 2019, from https://www.dummies.com/food-drink/recipes/a-brief-history-of-juicing/

The Full History of Juicing: Is it Just a Trend? - Well Pared | Billings, MT. (2018, January 26). Retrieved October 28, 2019, from https://wellpared.com/full-history-juicing-not-trend/

Crocker, P. (2016b, March 26). What You Can't Juice - dummies. Retrieved October 29, 2019, from https://www.dummies.com/food-drink/recipes/what-you-cant-juice/

Butler, N. (2018, December 3). Juicing vs. Blending: Which Is Better for Me? Retrieved November 2, 2019, from https://www.healthline.com/health/food-nutrition/juicing-vs-blending

Leech, J. (2017, June 4). Good Fiber, Bad Fiber - How The Different Types Affect You. Retrieved November 2, 2019, from https://www.healthline.com/nutrition/different-types-of-fiber#section7

Huizen, J. (2017, August 31). Soluble and insoluble fiber: What is the difference? Retrieved November 2, 2019, from https://www.medicalnewstoday.com/articles/319176.php

Carr, K. (2018, December 21). How to Choose the Best Juicer. Retrieved November 2, 2019, from https://kriscarr.com/blog/how-to-choose-best-juicer/

Picincu, A. (2019, June 24). 30-Day Juice Diet. Retrieved November 2, 2019, from https://www.livestrong.com/article/319561-30-day-juice-diet/

30 Day Juice Fast For Weight Loss Ultimate Guide. (2019, February 18). Retrieved November 2, 2019, from https://bestjuiceforweightloss.com/30-day-juice-fast-weight-loss/

Fogoros, R. (2019, September 10). What Is a Detox Diet? Retrieved November 4, 2019, from https://www.verywellfit.com/the-one-week-detox-diet-88250

Fogoros, R. (2019a, June 25). What Is a Juice Cleanse? Retrieved November 4, 2019, from https://www.verywellfit.com/juice-cleanse-89120

Voo, J. (n.d.). https://www.shape.com. Retrieved November 4, 2019, from https://www.shape.com/healthy-eating/healthy-drinks/10-green-smoothies-anyone-will-love?slide=c0ef022f-0424-428e-9505-5e8de7bf4ccb#c0ef022f-0424-428e-9505-5e8de7bf4ccb

Young, M. (2019, September 26). The Ultimate Guide To Juice Cleansing – Everything You Need To Know for Beginners, Weight Loss, DIY and More. Retrieved November 4, 2019, from https://www.juicebuff.com/juice-cleanse-weight-loss/

Burton, N. (2018, November 30). The Hidden Dangers of Juicing. Retrieved November 4, 2019, from https://stylecaster.com/beauty/the-hidden-dangers-of-juicing/

Nall, R. (2018b, September 21). What are the pros and cons of a juice cleanse? Retrieved November 4, 2019, from https://www.medicalnewstoday.com/articles/323136.php

Hannum, R. (2019, October 1). How to Avoid the 5 Dangers of Juicing and Smoothies. Retrieved November 4, 2019, from https://www.thespruceeats.com/avoid-dangers-of-juicing-and-smoothies-2078418

Arnarson, A. (2019, May 8). Apples 101: Nutrition Facts and Health Benefits. Retrieved October 28, 2019, from https://www.healthline.com/nutrition/foods/apples#benefits

Davidson, K. (2019, June 5). 9 Health and Nutrition Benefits of Apricots. Retrieved November 2, 2019, from https://www.healthline.com/nutrition/apricots-benefits#section7

Nutrition Facts For Apricots. (n.d.). Retrieved November 2, 2019, from https://tools.myfooddata.com/nutrition-facts.php?food=9021&serv=wt1

Cervoni, B. (2019, October 14). Blackberries Nutrition Facts. Retrieved November 4, 2019, from https://www.verywellfit.com/blackberry-nutrition-facts-calories-and-health-benefits-4109221

McDermott, A. (2017, July 14). Blackberries: Health Benefits and Nutrition Information. Retrieved November 4, 2019, from https://www.healthline.com/health/benefits-of-blackberries

Palsdottir, H. (2019, February 20). Blueberries 101: Nutrition Facts and Health Benefits. Retrieved November 4, 2019, from https://www.healthline.com/nutrition/foods/blueberries

McDermott, A. (2019, October 11). 7 Nutritious Benefits of Eating Cantaloupe. Retrieved November 4, 2019, from https://www.healthline.com/health/food-nutrition/benefits-of-cantaloupe#how-to-choose-cantaloupe

Elliott, B. (2017, February 18). 10 Science-Based Benefits of Grapefruit. Retrieved November 4, 2019, from https://www.healthline.com/nutrition/10-benefits-of-grapefruit#section5

Groves, M. (2018, August 22). Top 12 Health Benefits of Eating Grapes. Retrieved November 4, 2019, from https://www.healthline.com/nutrition/benefits-of-grapes

Bjarnadottir, A. (2019, March 22). Lemons 101: Nutrition Facts and Health Benefits. Retrieved November 4, 2019, from https://www.healthline.com/nutrition/foods/lemons#vitamins-and-minerals

Raman, R. (2018, December 17). Mango: Nutrition, Health Benefits and How to Eat It. Retrieved November 4, 2019, from https://www.healthline.com/nutrition/mango

Arnarson, A. (2019, March 18). Oranges 101: Nutrition Facts and Health Benefits. Retrieved November 4, 2019, from https://www.healthline.com/nutrition/foods/oranges

Spritzler, F. (2018, December 4). 8 Evidence-Based Health Benefits of Papaya. Retrieved November 4, 2019, from https://www.healthline.com/nutrition/8-proven-papaya-benefits#section1

Petre, A. (2019, January 17). 10 Surprising Health Benefits and Uses of Peaches. Retrieved November 4, 2019, from https://www.healthline.com/nutrition/peach-fruit-benefits

Cervoni, B. (2019, October 14). Pear Nutrition Facts. Retrieved November 4, 2019, from https://www.verywellfit.com/pears-nutrition-facts-calories-and-health-benefits-4114350

Raman, R. (2018, May 26). 8 Impressive Health Benefits of Pineapple. Retrieved November 4, 2019, from https://www.healthline.com/nutrition/benefits-of-pineapple#section1

Elliott, B. (2017, May 13). 7 Health Benefits of Plums and Prunes. Retrieved November 4, 2019, from https://www.healthline.com/nutrition/benefits-of-plums-prunes

Groves, M. (2018, October 13). Red Raspberries: Nutrition Facts, Benefits and More. Retrieved November 4, 2019, from https://www.healthline.com/nutrition/raspberry-nutrition

Bjarnadottir, A. (2019, March 27). Strawberries 101: Nutrition Facts and Health Benefits. Retrieved November 4, 2019, from https://www.healthline.com/nutrition/foods/strawberries#nutrition

Bjarnadottir, A. (2019a, March 25). Tomatoes 101: Nutrition Facts and Health Benefits. Retrieved November 4, 2019, from https://www.healthline.com/nutrition/foods/tomatoes

17 Fruits Highest in Water. (2019, October 14). Retrieved November 4, 2019, from https://www.myfooddata.com/articles/fruits-high-in-water.php

Coyle, D. (2018, April 4). 7 Reasons Why You Should Eat More Asparagus. Retrieved November 4, 2019, from https://www.healthline.com/nutrition/asparagus-benefits#section2

Bjarnadottir, A. (2019, March 8). Beetroot 101: Nutrition Facts and Health Benefits. Retrieved November 4, 2019, from https://www.healthline.com/nutrition/foods/beetroot#nutrition

McDermott, A. (2018, September 18). 12 Health Benefits of Beetroot Juice. Retrieved November 4, 2019, from https://www.healthline.com/health/food-nutrition/beetroot-juice-benefits#slow-dementia

Arnarson, A. (2019, March 27). Bell Peppers 101: Nutrition Facts and Health Benefits. Retrieved November 4, 2019, from https://www.healthline.com/nutrition/foods/bell-peppers

Enloe, A. (2018, July 1). The 13 Healthiest Leafy Green Vegetables. Retrieved November 4, 2019, from https://www.healthline.com/nutrition/leafy-green-vegetables#section10

Bjarnadottir, A. (2019c, May 10). Broccoli 101: Nutrition Facts and Health Benefits. Retrieved November 4, 2019, from https://www.healthline.com/nutrition/foods/broccoli

Kubala, J. (2017, November 4). 9 Impressive Health Benefits of Cabbage. Retrieved November 4, 2019, from https://www.healthline.com/nutrition/benefits-of-cabbage

Bjarnadottir, A. (2019c, May 3). Carrots 101: Nutrition Facts and Health Benefits. Retrieved November 4, 2019, from https://www.healthline.com/nutrition/foods/carrots#organic

Elliott, B. (2017, April 14). The Top 8 Health Benefits of Cauliflower. Retrieved November 4, 2019, from https://www.healthline.com/nutrition/benefits-of-cauliflower

Cronkleton, E. (2018, August 14). Benefits of Celery Juice. Retrieved November 4, 2019, from https://www.healthline.com/health/celery-juice#recipe

Berkheiser, K. (2019, June 4). 9 Health and Nutrition Benefits of Red Leaf Lettuce. Retrieved November 4, 2019, from https://www.healthline.com/nutrition/red-leaf-lettuce

Bjarnadottir, A. (2019d, May 8). Onions 101: Nutrition Facts and Health Effects. Retrieved November 4, 2019, from https://www.healthline.com/nutrition/foods/onions

Arnarson, A. (2019a, March 7). Potatoes 101: Nutrition Facts and Health Effects. Retrieved November 4, 2019, from https://www.healthline.com/nutrition/foods/potatoes#nutrition

Jennings, K. (2016, December 26). Pumpkin: Nutrition, Benefits and How to Eat. Retrieved November 4, 2019, from https://www.healthline.com/nutrition/pumpkin-nutrition-review#section4

McDermott, A. (2018, May 18). Are Radishes Good for You? Retrieved November 4, 2019, from https://www.healthline.com/health/food-nutrition/the-benefits-of-radishes#1

Gunnars, K. (2019, May 14). Spinach 101: Nutrition Facts and Health Benefits. Retrieved November 4, 2019, from https://www.healthline.com/nutrition/foods/spinach#benefits

Bjarnadottir, A. (2019, May 13). Sweet Potatoes 101: Nutrition Facts and Health Benefits. Retrieved November 4, 2019, from https://www.healthline.com/nutrition/foods/sweet-potatoes

Kubala, J. (2018, December 4). Swiss Chard: Nutrition, Benefits and How to Cook It. Retrieved November 4, 2019, from https://www.healthline.com/nutrition/swiss-chard

Groves, M. (2018, August 6). 10 Impressive Health Benefits of Watercress. Retrieved November 4, 2019, from https://www.healthline.com/nutrition/watercress-benefits

Petre, A. (2019, February 19). 12 Health and Nutrition Benefits of Zucchini. Retrieved November 4, 2019, from https://www.healthline.com/nutrition/zucchini-benefits

17 Vegetables Highest in Water. (2019, October 14). Retrieved November 4, 2019, from https://www.myfooddata.com/articles/vegetables-high-in-water.php

Picincu, A. (2019, July 5). How to Ease Out of a Juice Fast. Retrieved November 4, 2019, from https://www.livestrong.com/article/546063-how-to-ease-out-of-a-juice-fast/

Wong, C. (2019, March 11). The Right and Safe Way to Ending a Cleanse. Retrieved November 4, 2019, from https://www.verywellfit.com/how-to-end-a-cleanse-89112

Nall, R. (2018, September 21). What are the pros and cons of a juice cleanse? Retrieved November 4, 2019, from https://www.medicalnewstoday.com/articles/323136.php

Waring, S. (2014, March 18). Getting back to normal, post-cleanse tips & tricks. Retrieved November 4, 2019, from https://www.juicenashville.com/blogs/news/12728313-getting-back-to-normal-post-cleanse-tips-tricks

Claim your FREE Audiobook Now

Autoimmune Healing Transform Your Health, Reduce Inflammation, Heal the Immune System and Start Living Healthy

Do you have an overall sense of not feeling your best, but it has been going on so long that it's actually normal to you?

If you answered yes to any of these question, you may have an autoimmune disease.

Autoimmune diseases are one of the ten leading causes of death for women in all age groups and they affect nearly 25 million Americans.

In fact millions of people worldwide suffer from autoimmunity whether they know it or not.

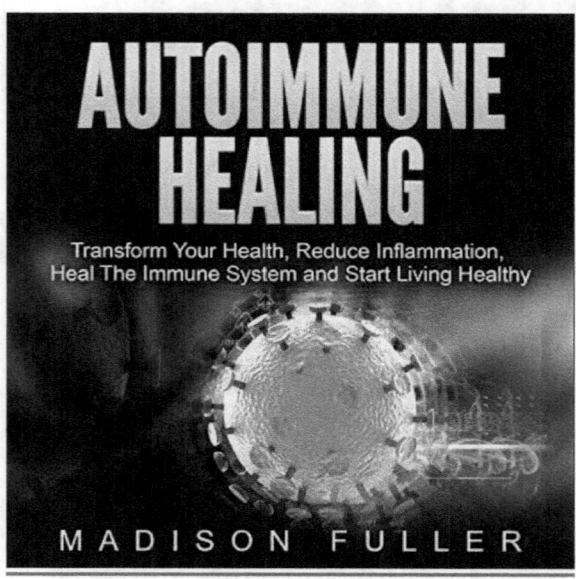

Want More?

Health, longevity and lifestyle tips and advice

Sign up to get the exclusive Madison Fuller e-newsletter, sent out every week

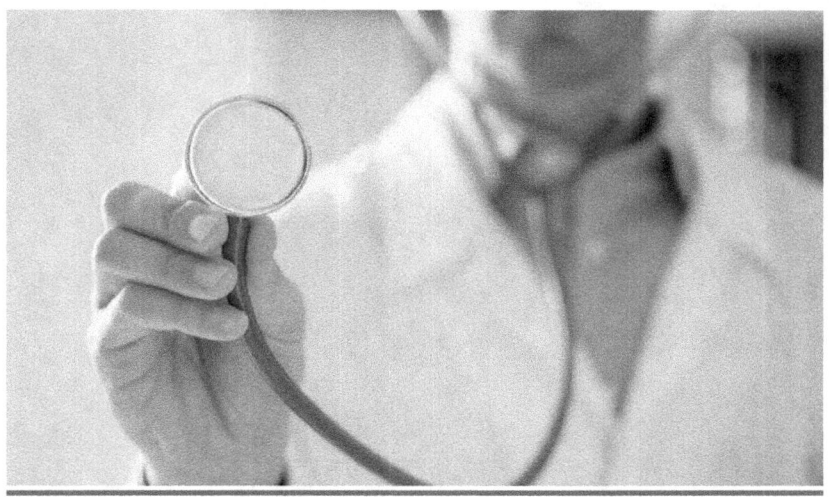

https://www.subscribepage.com/autoimmune

www.ingramcontent.com/pod-product-compliance
Lightning Source LLC
Chambersburg PA
CBHW071230080526
44587CB00013BA/1553